The FORTY FIX

The Real-World Guide to Fat Loss, Hormone Shifts, and Feeling Like Yourself Again After 40

Aimee Meier & Erica Jennings

The Forty Fix

The Real-World Guide to Fat Loss, Hormone Shifts, and Feeling Like Yourself Again After 40

Aimee Meier & Erica Jennings

Soulfuential Publishing helps female coaches, creators, and entrepreneurs increase their impact and grow emotional connections with their audience via the world's most powerful medium - books. Learn more at soulfuential.com

Disclaimer

The information and insights shared in this book are based on the authors' personal experiences and perspectives. The content is intended for informational and inspirational purposes only and should not be considered a substitute for professional medical advice, diagnosis, or treatment.

The authors are not licensed mental health professionals, therapists, or medical doctors. Always seek the advice of your physician, therapist, or other qualified health provider with any questions you may have regarding a mental health or medical condition. Never disregard professional advice or delay seeking it because of something you have read in this book.

Table of Contents

For You

If you're holding this book in your hands (or scrolling through it on your phone), you're probably looking for a better way. Maybe you've tried every plan, every program, every calorie-counting app and still feel stuck in a body that doesn't feel like yours. Maybe you've spent years putting everyone else first, and now your body is waving the white flag. Or maybe, like the two of us, you've hit your forties and realized that what used to work . . . well, it just doesn't anymore.

You're not alone. And even more important? You're not doing anything wrong.

We know what it feels like to look in the mirror and not recognize the woman staring back. We know what it feels like to be told, "This is just how it is now," and feel defeated by that. We know how overwhelming it can be to try to figure out what your body actually *needs*—especially when the advice out there is all over the place. Low carb, no fat, fasted cardio, intermittent fasting, green juice, eat every three hours, skip breakfast, track your macros, count your calories, cleanse, restrict, reset . . . enough already.

Fix It In Your Favor

The Forty Fix is a declaration to start working with your body instead of against it. That's why we created The 100-50 Method. It started with a simple shift: instead of focusing on what to cut out, we asked: "What if we started adding in what our bodies are truly craving? What if we gave our bodies the nourishment, rhythm, and support they've been quietly asking for all along?"

This method isn't a crash diet or a thirty-day challenge. It's a sustainable rhythm for real women in real life. Women who are juggling careers, kids, stress, hormones, and responsibilities and want to feel good in their bodies. We built this system with women like you in mind, and because we are women like you.

Who This Book Is For

This book is for the woman stepping into her forties and every year beyond.

For the woman who wakes up one morning and swears her body has changed overnight. For the woman who realizes the meals, the workouts, the "rules" that once worked just don't anymore.

Because what served you in the past belonged to a different season, a different body, a different time. This is for the woman who still wants weight loss, but not at the expense of her energy, her joy, or her life.

She wants a fix that fits now.

A way forward that works with her body, not against it. It's for the woman ready to release extremes, to stop chasing quick fixes, and to finally build results that last because they're rooted in alignment, not restriction.

This is your freedom era.
Your I-get-to-feel-good-again era.
Your this-time-it's-sustainable era.

Weight loss in your forties isn't about doing less.

It's about living more fully in the body you were made to thrive in.

Is This Still For Me If...

One of the most common questions we get is, "Can I do this if I'm a vegetarian or vegan?" And the answer? A resounding YES! Every woman, no matter her dietary preferences, needs 100 grams of protein and 50 grams of healthy fats daily to properly fuel her body. We'll show you exactly how to make it happen.

Another big question: "Is this method helpful if I'm taking GLP-1 medication for weight loss or microdosing for longevity?" Again, a big YES. In fact, it's essential for women using peptides to incorporate these strategies to maintain muscle mass, strength, and overall health while on their weight loss journey.

At the end of the day, this method is for all women. It's our heartfelt mission to help you step into better health through a simple and sustainable system, so you can show up in every other part of life as the best version of yourself.

What You Will Gain from This Book

Inside this book, we'll walk you through a method that's helped us (and now thousands of others) reclaim energy, balance hormones, and finally feel in control again. You'll learn the science-backed strategy behind why this works and get practical, real-life tools to help you make it your own. We'll also share our personal stories, the setbacks and breakthroughs, and the habits that changed everything for us.

But more than anything, we hope this book gives you something even more powerful than a meal plan: *hope*. A renewed sense of possibility. A belief that it's never too late to feel like yourself again (or maybe even better than you've ever felt) so you can show up in every other part of life as the best version of yourself.

That hope is so important because, just like us, you were probably told somewhere along the line that our bodies were supposed to "slow down" after forty. That energy would fade, hormones would rage, and our jeans would just magically shrink. That once we crossed into this new decade, we were supposed to settle for less. Less energy, less confidence, and maybe even less of ourselves.

We Call BS on "It's All Downhill After Forty"

The Forty Fix was born out of a deep desire to rewrite that story. We didn't "bounce back." We came back stronger, more grounded, and more ourselves. No magic pills, no quick fixes, just real ways to move, fuel, and show up fully in this season.

They say things start to fall apart at forty. We call BS. Not only that, but this book is made to flip the script and fix it in our favor.

So whether you're just starting out or already halfway in, we're so glad you're here. Let's dive in and get started.

Because this?

This is for you.

The Year We Turned Forty

Hi, we're Aimee and Erica! We're two busy working moms who've been through the ups and downs of midlife weight gain, hormonal shifts, and all the challenges that come with this season of life. After navigating it ourselves, we created The 100-50 Method to help women like you feel your absolute best, inside and out.

Let's go back to a few years ago. This was us then. (February & June of 2022).

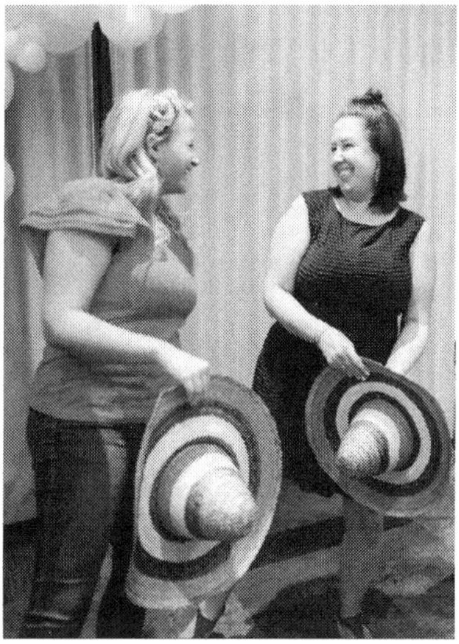

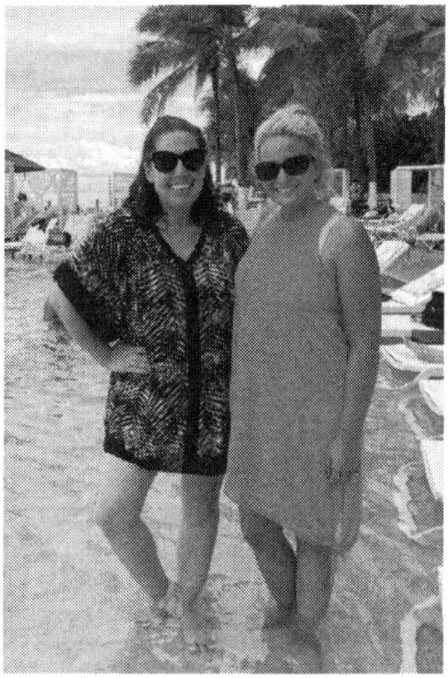

The Day the Couch Became Gravitron

Aimee's Story

It was 9:00 a.m. on Saturday morning, and there I was: stuck on the couch, feeling utterly drained. Imagine being on that favorite '80s fair ride, the Gravitron, where you're spun so fast you feel pinned against the wall. That was me. I didn't have the strength in my bones to lift a limb from the gravitational force keeping it glued to the couch. Meanwhile, the chaos played out around me.

My five kids were unleashing their Saturday-morning energy: laughing, squabbling, chasing each other from room to room, celebrating, dancing, and screaming with joy . . . until a stolen toy, a spilled snack, or a minor fall turned those joyful shouts into cries of frustration.

And me? I barely registered any of it. I had drifted off to sleep on the couch while flames swirled around me.

Gosh, do I wish I could say this was a one-off occurrence.

But it wasn't.

This was a typical weekend morning.

At forty, I was waking up every morning feeling exhausted. And every time I reached for a little food to boost my energy, I somehow ended up feeling even more drowsy.

"How am I always so tired? How did I get here?" I wondered on this particular November morning.

After five beautiful daughters and a twin delivery at age thirty-eight that pushed me past my limits, I found myself locked in an uphill battle with hormonal weight.

By the time my youngest ones hit their second birthday (and I hit my forties), my energy was nearly non-existent, my sugar cravings were overwhelming, and I was carrying an extra seventy-five pounds, especially around my midsection, that wouldn't budge despite my best efforts.

For years, I confided in health professionals about my constant exhaustion, insatiable cravings for sugar and carbs, and tiredness throughout the day, even after a full night's sleep.

I was told it was normal: "That's just what happens in your forties." "You have five kids. It's a lot." "You have autistic twins. It's exhausting."

Oh, and the other thing I heard a lot: "That's pretty typical for women with PCOS."

Yup, my entire adult life, I struggled with polycystic ovary syndrome (PCOS) and all the frustrating, painful symptoms that come along with it, including needing medical interventions just to grow our family.

The thing I never once heard from a medical professional: "Did you know your nutrition might be the key to all of this?"

No one ever mentioned how it was even possible my nutrition was contributing to my struggles. No one told me about the importance of blood sugar balance. No one ever sat me down to explain the benefits of eating for your insulin hormone.

Yes, I knew I should be eating better. Yes, I knew I should be nourishing my body better.

BUT the idea that food alone could be key to it all never crossed my mind.

Everything changed when I decided to flip the script. Instead of obsessing over what to cut out, I started focusing on what to add. I began intentionally incorporating nutrient-rich foods that balanced my hormones.

Nourishing my body in a way that balanced my hormones was completely new to me.

Slowly but surely, my cravings started to fade, my sleep improved dramatically, and my energy levels soared. Over time, my PCOS symptoms eased, my depression lifted, and those stubborn extra seventy-five pounds melted away.

This transformation started the steps and habits that would become The 100-50 Method, a system that will teach you how to truly fuel your body without the endless cycle of deprivation.

If you've ever felt trapped in a loop of fatigue, sugar crashes, and weight that just won't shift, know that you're not alone.

In fact, while I was hitting rock bottom at age forty, my dear friend Erica was on a similar journey, facing her own set of challenges.

My Lowest Low at The Happiest Place On Earth

Erica's Story

I remember the day clearly, August 3, 2022. I was in Orlando, Florida, for a work convention, and every outfit I had was tight. Nothing fit the way it used to. I felt like my body was just . . . different. I was sweating more than usual, and the tightness of my clothes made me feel suffocated, like I couldn't breathe freely.

Every time I looked in the mirror, I saw the weight, not just on my belly or stomach, but everywhere. My arms felt heavier, my thighs rubbed together, and I could see my face was fuller, rounder. I hated every picture that was taken of me that weekend. I cringed when I saw myself, not because I didn't like the woman staring back at me, but because I didn't recognize her. I felt embarrassed, almost as if I had failed somehow. The weight felt suffocating, and I couldn't shake the feeling that my body had betrayed me. I found myself constantly adjusting my clothes, pulling at the fabric to make it less tight, trying to hide the rolls that were now there. I was so uncomfortable in my own skin. I remember trying to hide in work photos, not wanting to be seen, wishing I could just disappear from the frame.

I was thirty-nine years old, and I just couldn't figure out what was happening to my body.

Earlier that summer, in May, I had started noticing my weight creeping up, and fast. It felt like it came out of nowhere. I was doing everything I was "supposed to" be doing: going to Orangetheory five times a week, pushing myself to the limit to rack up splat points, thinking the only way to lose the belly was to run myself crazy there. But no matter what, nothing was changing. My bra line bulge wouldn't go away, I was gaining weight in my chest, and my face was constantly inflamed. I was eating "clean," I wasn't indulging in nightly wine or junk food, and yet the scale kept going up. I was beyond frustrated. I felt like my body was betraying me.

I decided to go to the doctor, thinking maybe my thyroid was "off," like I had heard many women say. But when the tests came back, my hormones were normal. I couldn't understand it. It was like my body had just turned on me. I met with a trainer at the gym, hoping that maybe personal training would kickstart something. I remember stepping on the Body Scan and seeing my BMI was 38 percent, and I was at my heaviest weight of 168 pounds. I was in shock. I felt hopeless. It didn't make sense. I had been through pregnancy and post-partum before and lost the weight, but this time . . . it just wasn't happening.

I was doing all the right things, but nothing seemed to work. As the summer went on, I started hearing about Ozempic from a friend. She was seeing great results, and I thought, "Maybe that's it. Maybe that's the magic I need to lose this weight." Desperate, I applied for the medication, thinking it would be my last resort. But I was denied. It felt like the door had closed before I even had a chance to try.

That moment hit me hard. I thought, "What now?" I was at my wit's end, stuck in a cycle of frustration and confusion. But it was at that very moment, feeling totally helpless and defeated, that I had my breakthrough.

I remember having an aha moment looking at my lab results and specifically my insulin fasting numbers. I had a history of gestational diabetes during my pregnancies, and that experience had left me hyper-aware of how my body responded to weight and insulin levels. When I was pregnant, I had to monitor my blood sugar levels constantly, which was a terrifying and exhausting experience. I remember the strict diet, the endless finger pricks, and the constant worry about whether my blood sugar levels were too high or too low. I had to be so careful about everything I ate, making sure I didn't slip up and risk my health or my baby's. It was stressful, and it felt like I was always walking a fine line. I was relieved when my pregnancies ended, thinking that once the baby was born, everything would go back to normal.

But even after giving birth, the effects of gestational diabetes lingered in ways I hadn't anticipated. I knew I was at a higher risk for developing type 2 diabetes down the road, so I had to be vigilant about maintaining a healthy weight and eating balanced meals. But this time, I couldn't understand what was going on. I had managed my health so carefully after pregnancy, but the weight gain I was experiencing now at almost forty felt completely out of my control.

It wasn't just a few extra pounds; it felt like my body was in revolt. No matter how much I exercised, ate clean, or stuck to what had worked for me in the past, my body kept changing in ways that were frustrating. Why didn't anyone mention that weight gain at forty is REAL!

Our two stories have led us to this.

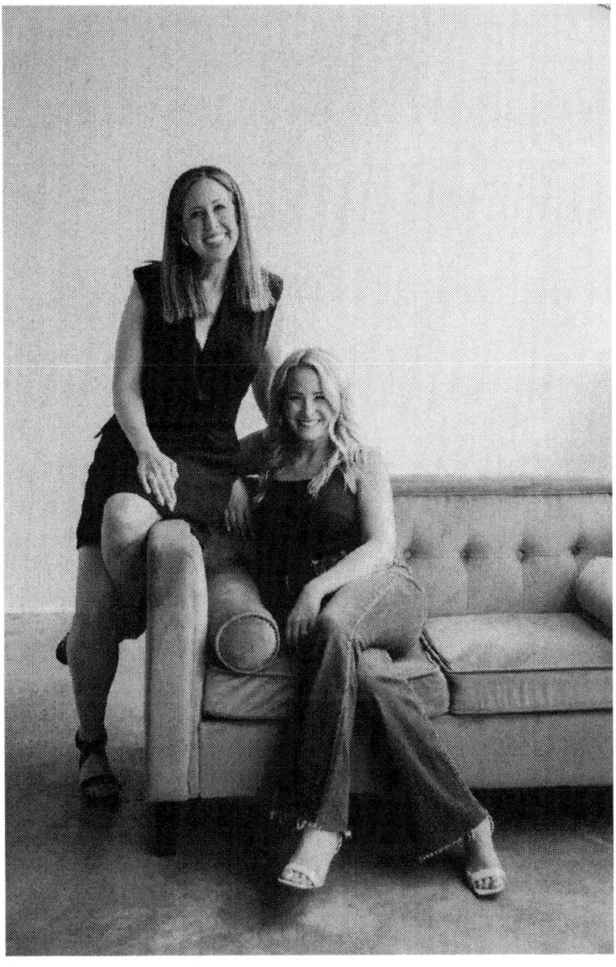

These are the experiences that brought us right here, to what we now call The 100-50 Method. It all started with a simple desire to feel better, nourish our bodies, lose weight, and kick that sluggish energy. And honestly? Just to feel good again. Along the way, we found so many unexpected benefits that we couldn't keep to ourselves.

Let's hit pause for a second though. This method comes from our own experiences, and while we're excited to share it with you, always listen to your body and consult with a healthcare professional if you have any concerns or questions.

You've heard our stories, and we want to be really clear: we're not doctors, nutritionists, or dietitians. We're two moms in our forties who, after feeling the weight of hormonal changes (literally and figuratively), decided to make simple, sustainable changes that actually worked. With years of experience in the wellness space, we've learned what truly makes a difference. We created a system that's easy to remember. No complicated tracking. No feeling like you need to be an expert or have a PhD to dissect everything. Just real food, practical habits, and a method that fuels our bodies so we can show up as our best selves in all the other roles we play.

And once we started feeling the difference? Friends and family noticed. They asked, "What are you doing?" And we found ourselves sharing this simple approach over and over. Eventually, it became a catchphrase between us: The 100-50 Method. Because that's how it all began, adding in whole foods to hit 100 grams of protein and 50 grams of healthy fats each day.

Of course, there were a few other simple shifts along the way. And those shifts became the foundation for what we now call M.E.T.H.O.D., an easy-to-remember roadmap we've created to help other women, just like us, thrive and feel their best.

Now, we're passing it on to you. In the next few chapters, we'll walk you through this simple, doable strategy that can help you create a sustainable, feel-good lifestyle as you move through your forties and beyond.

M.E.T.H.O.D.

The 100-50 Method isn't another quick-fix diet. It is the proven system behind *The Forty Fix*, a sustainable way to reset your energy, support your hormones, and reach your weight loss goals by working *with* your body, not against it. It's rooted in simple, powerful principles: nourish with purpose and lean into your body's natural rhythms.

In the chapters ahead, we'll dive into everything from balanced macros and quick exercise snacks to a simple three-meals-a-day routine, all while focusing on your hormonal health. We'll share daily practices that help you keep moving forward. By making small, intentional changes each day, you'll set yourself up for lasting, transformative results.

We like to keep things simple and easy to remember so they actually stick, right?

So here's an easy little acronym for what we'll be diving into throughout this book: M.E.T.H.O.D. Let's break it down together!

M – Macros

E – Exercise Snacks

T – Three Meals a Day

H – Hormones

O – Optimization

D – Daily

We truly believe the tools and strategies in this book can help you create the vibrant, balanced life you've been craving. Whether you're navigating postpartum changes, dealing with hormonal shifts at midlife, or just ready to embrace a healthier lifestyle, The 100-50 Method is here to support you every step of the way.

Let's jump in and start this journey together: toward more energy, balanced hormones, and a life full of vitality!

Chapter 1

M: Macros

Welcome to the very first pillar of The 100-50 Method: **Macros.** This is the foundation of *The Forty Fix*, the place where lasting change begins. Before your mind starts racing to endless calorie counting and complicated nutrition charts, let's hit pause and simplify things.

In this method, we're focusing on just two essential macros: **protein** and **healthy fats.**

Think of them as your nutritional power duo: nourishing, balancing, and totally in sync with your body's natural rhythm.

Why 100 Grams of Protein and 50 Grams of Healthy Fats? Let's Talk Macros

When we talk about *macros*, we're usually breaking it down into protein, fats, and carbs. But here's the deal, The 100-50 Method isn't about obsessing over every single macro. Instead, it's about focusing on what your body actually needs more of. Protein and healthy fats are the two most important macros for fat loss and keeping your body in fat-burning mode. That's why we zero in on **100 grams of protein and 50 grams of healthy fats** every single day.

Why?

1. Because when women come to us, these are the two nutrients they're usually not getting enough of.

2. We know this because we weren't eating nearly enough of them when our whole journey with hormonal weight gain started.

3. And most importantly, because protein and healthy fats are the key players in keeping your blood sugar stable, supporting insulin, and getting off the constant craving rollercoaster.

This method is all about what to *ADD IN* to your meals so you feel *full*, fueled, and balanced. Most of the women we work with are either eating way too little or grazing all day without actually nourishing their bodies. Sound familiar?

Some women come in barely eating enough to function, maybe skipping breakfast, surviving on coffee, grabbing a late lunch, and then barely having a real meal for dinner . . . and yet, somehow, the weight still won't budge.

Other women are eating all day long. They start with Starbucks for breakfast, grab a working lunch, snack on granola and yogurt at 3:00 p.m., have dinner with the family, and then binge once the kids go to bed. Even though they're eating a ton of calories, their bodies are still craving more because they're undernourished in protein and healthy fats.

Do either of those sound like you? If so, you're not alone. And that's exactly why this method works. It's about giving your body what it *actually* needs so you can break free from the cycle and finally feel in control again.

Why Protein and Healthy Fats? The Two Pillars of The 100-50 Method

Protein: Your Body's Building Block

Protein isn't just about muscle. Confession: growing up, I was the girl who thought protein shakes were just for bodybuilders, and therefore not for me.

Now, in a time where protein is praised and talked about constantly, we hear about protein for all the useful ways it's used in our body. It repairs, rebuilds, and rejuvenates.

It's the foundation for nearly everything your body does. From repairing tissues and supporting hormone production to keeping your hair, skin, and nails healthy, protein is your body's behind-the-scenes powerhouse. It's made of amino acids, which are essential for rebuilding and maintaining everything from your muscles to your metabolism.

And when you're eating enough of it consistently, it makes a noticeable difference, not just in how you look, but in how you *feel.*

One of the biggest benefits of prioritizing protein is how it helps you stay full and satisfied. It naturally curbs cravings, balances blood sugar, and keeps your energy steady between meals.

Plus, your body actually burns more calories digesting protein than it does carbs or fat. That's right, just eating it gives your metabolism a boost.

When you focus on eating at least 100 grams of protein a day as part of The 100-50 Method, you're giving your body the steady fuel it needs to function at its best.

Healthy Fats: The Unsung Hero

With 50 grams of healthy fats daily, you're setting the stage for stable blood sugar levels and a happy, balanced insulin response. Think of healthy fats as the calming influence that keeps your energy (and your mood) in check.

If you lived through the '90s (especially if you were a kid or teen like we were), you probably remember being told that fat was the enemy. We were told that fat was the thing making us gain weight. Gosh, we were so misled!

The truth is, healthy fats are essential for healthy bodies. They help support hormone production, which is key for everything from metabolism to mood. Plus, fats are necessary for absorbing important vitamins like A, D, E, and K, which are vital for things like bone health and immunity.

Here's the real kicker: healthy fats provide long-lasting energy that keeps us feeling full and steady, instead of riding the blood sugar roller coaster that leads to cravings.

When we eat healthy fats (think avocados, nuts, olive oil, and fatty fish), our bodies break them down into fatty acids and glycerol, which are used to produce energy and build cell membranes.

Fats also help make hormones like estrogen and testosterone, which play a huge role in balancing everything, especially as we go through changes like perimenopause or menopause. So, far from being the villain, healthy fats are actually the unsung heroes that help keep us balanced, energized, and feeling our best.

Why Protein & Healthy Fats Help GLUCOSE SPIKES

When going all in with The 100-50 Method, it's key to understand what glucose spikes are and how they affect your body.

Stabilizing blood sugar is important when it comes to balanced hormones, sustained energy, and effortless fat loss.

Under normal circumstances, your blood sugar rises gradually after a meal and then steadily returns to baseline. Glucose spikes are different. They happen when you consume something that causes your blood sugar to surge so quickly that your body overcorrects, leading to a sudden crash, dropping even lower than where you started. It's the difference between riding a gentle wave (stable) and being whipped around on a rollercoaster (spikey).

Glucose spikes can cause energy crashes and cravings and can negatively impact your sleep, energy, mood, and focus. Consistent glucose spikes can also lead to health complications such as insulin resistance, type 2 diabetes, and heart disease.

Here is what's going on in your body when your blood sugar is out of balance, and why that matters.

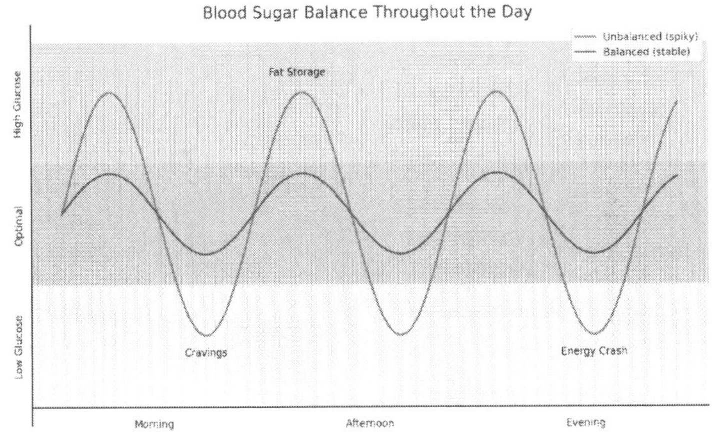

The graph above shows two different patterns: The red line represents a typical "rollercoaster day" where blood sugar spikes high after meals (often carb-heavy or sugary ones), then crashes down, leaving you feeling tired, moody, and craving more sugar. This up-and-down pattern can wreak havoc on your energy, hormones, and fat storage.

Now compare that to the green line. This is what we aim for with The 100-50 Method. Instead of big highs and lows, your blood sugar stays within an ideal range. It remains stable, steady, and supportive of long-term health. This stability is what helps your insulin levels normalize, your GLP-1 hormone stay active, and your body stay in fat-burning mode without the crash-and-burn cycle.

When you avoid those wild spikes, you're not just dodging energy crashes, but you're also keeping insulin in check, reducing cravings, and creating the ideal environment for your body to burn fat instead of storing it.

This isn't just about *what* we eat, but *how* those foods impact our blood sugar, hormones, and metabolism. That's why protein and healthy fats are the foundation. They keep us full, fueled, and in fat-burning mode all day long.

When we eat high-carb or sugary foods, our blood sugar shoots up fast, triggering a big insulin release. And while insulin's just doing its job (bringing that sugar back down), those constant spikes and crashes leave us feeling sluggish, hungrier, and stuck in a cycle that makes fat loss harder.

That's why **protein and healthy fats** are the foundation of The 100-50 Method. They keep blood sugar levels steady, helping with energy, satiety, and hormone balance.

Why We Don't Count Calories or Other Macros

Here's the real talk: forget about obsessing over every calorie. That "calories in, calories out" mantra from the 1980s is a myth, especially when your hormones are out of whack.

The typical Instagram fitness bros will have you believe that restriction is the path to weight loss, but that's where the truth gets lost in the noise.

When you're undernourished and your hormones are out of whack, that's simply not the case.

Plus, you're more likely to binge when focused on restriction, and that constant cycle of deprivation only makes things worse.

In The 100-50 Method, we choose whole, nutrient-dense foods. We're not playing a numbers game with calories; we're focusing on nourishment.

When you feed your body well with protein and healthy fats, you naturally curb those hunger pangs. You more easily keep your blood sugar balanced, and your body lets the weight drop without always feeling deprived. Your energy starts to go up, your inflammation starts to go down, and you get off the glucose rollercoaster. This method is about fueling your body, not punishing it.

Practical Tips for Balancing Protein and Healthy Fats

Daily Targets Made Simple

- **100g of Protein:** Incorporate sources like lean meats, eggs, legumes, or even a protein shake if you need that extra boost.
- **50g of Healthy Fats:** Think avocados, nuts, seeds, olive oil, foods that not only taste great but also work wonders for your hormonal balance.

Meal-Planning Strategies

The following are the types of foods you will base your meals around:

- **Omega-3s:** Incorporate salmon or mackerel for omega-3s and healthy fats.
- **Avocados:** Add avocado to meals or snacks for healthy fats and fiber.
- **Seeds:** Sprinkle chia seeds, ground flax, or hemp seeds into your meals, smoothies, or yogurt.
- **Healthy oils:** Cook with olive, avocado, or coconut oil for better fats.
- **Plant proteins:** Use beans, lentils, and quinoa as protein-rich, plant-based options.

- **Full-fat dairy:** Choose grass-fed butter, cheese, or unsweetened Greek yogurt for protein and healthy fats.
- **Olives & coconut:** Snack on olives or use coconut products for healthy fats.
- **Lean meats:** Choose lean cuts of meat like chicken breast or turkey for protein.

Want to see some simple, real-life examples? At the end of this book, we've each shared our 7-day food journal, starting on page 127. And if you need a quick reference sheet, don't worry! We've got one for both protein and healthy fats at the end of this chapter to make it even easier for you.

Listen to Your Body

The beauty of this approach is that you're not stuck obsessing over calorie counts. Instead, you're learning to listen to your body. When you're properly nourished, you'll feel more energized, cravings become less of an issue, and you'll find that sweet spot where your mood and metabolism are in harmony.

Putting The Method Into Practice

Before you close this chapter, take a moment to reflect:

- **Set your daily targets:** Keep it simple with 100g of protein and 50g of healthy fats. These are the building blocks that fuel your body and keep you in fat-burning mode.

- **Plan your meals:** Use the suggestions above as a starting point. Experiment and find what makes you feel nourished and satisfied. In the "Three Meals a Day" chapter, we'll dive deeper into the tools that set you up for success.
- **Trust your body:** When you feed your body the right foods, it knows exactly what to do. No more calorie counting, no guilt, just real, sustainable fat-burning at forty and beyond.

This isn't another crash diet to try. It's a powerful shift in how you live. It's about honoring your body, balancing your hormones, and unlocking a fat-burning rhythm that works with you, not against you. Embrace it. Enjoy it. Watch your body transform as you take control of your health and your future.

Real Women, Real Wins

We've seen firsthand how this approach transforms lives. Here is what a few ladies we work with have said about macros and The 100-50 Method:

> "Tracking protein and fat seems so much easier than tracking and counting calories! It just 'feels' so much easier to do, but more importantly, so much easier to stay on track and figure out where you might need a little adjusting! I also think

a big takeaway was it's OK to eat, and there really aren't 'limitations.' You can adjust and finish the day up with at least 100/50 and still feel good about yourself! A lot of prior attempts at a new lifestyle and eating pattern/habits made me feel like I failed if I slipped up in one little spot! This is easier to adjust to and still stay on track!"
—Sara B.

"Upping my protein and fat has definitely helped me feel more full and prevent that 'hangry' feeling."
—Andrea R. B.

"Learning about macros shifted my mindset because I always thought it was too complicated to understand. What surprised me most was that I was eating nowhere near 100 grams of protein and 50 g of healthy fats a day. In fact, I was undereating the wrong foods, and when I did eat, the majority of my calories were in one meal because I was so hungry."
—Stephanie G.

Quick Protein Cheat Sheet:

Meat-Based Proteins (4 oz servings)

- Chicken breast – 32g protein
- Chicken thigh – 27g protein
- Turkey breast – 34g protein
- Ground beef (80% lean) – 19g protein
- Ground beef (90% lean) – 23g protein
- Ground beef (93% lean) – 24g protein
- Ground chicken – 20g protein
- Ground turkey (93% lean) – 21g protein
- Ground turkey (85% lean) – 19g protein
- Sirloin steak – 31g protein
- Pork tenderloin – 29g protein
- Ground pork – 19g protein

Fish and Seafood (4 oz servings, protein content adjusted)

- Salmon – 29g protein
- Tuna – 33g protein
- Cod – 27g protein
- Halibut – 21g protein
- Mahi-mahi – 29g protein
- Tilapia – 23g protein
- Shrimp – 27g protein

- Scallops – 23g protein
- Lobster – 25g protein
- Crab – 23g protein

Dairy and Eggs

- Greek yogurt (plain, nonfat, 1 cup) – 21g protein
- Cottage cheese (low-fat, 1/2 cup) – 14g protein
- Cheddar cheese (1 oz) – 7g protein
- Mozzarella cheese (1 oz) – 6g protein
- Parmesan cheese (1 oz) – 5g protein
- Swiss cheese (1 oz) – 8g protein
- Eggs (2 large) – 12g protein
- Egg whites (3 large) – 10g protein

Plant-Based Proteins

- Firm tofu (4 oz) – 11g protein
- Tempeh (4 oz) – 23g protein
- Edamame (1/2 cup) – 9g protein
- Lentils (1/2 cup) – 9g protein
- Chickpeas (1/2 cup) – 7g protein
- Black beans (1/2 cup) – 8g protein
- Lima beans (1/2 cup) – 6g protein
- Quinoa (1/2 cup) – 4g protein
- Hemp seeds (3 tbsp) – 10g protein
- Chia seeds (2 tbsp) – 4g protein

- Flax seeds (2 tbsp) – 3g protein
- Pumpkin seeds (1 oz) – 7g protein
- Sunflower seeds (1 oz) – 5g protein
- Almonds (1 oz) – 6g protein
- Walnuts (1 oz) – 4g protein
- Pecans (1 oz) – 3g protein
- Peanut butter (natural, 2 tbsp) – 8g protein
- Almond butter (2 tbsp) – 7g protein
- Seitan (4 oz) – 28g protein
- Nutritional yeast (2 tbsp) – 8g protein

Protein Powders (~30g serving)

- Whey protein powder – 25g protein
- Casein protein powder – 24g protein
- Soy protein powder – 20g protein
- Pea protein powder – 20g protein
- Hemp protein powder – 15g protein
- Brown rice protein powder – 18g protein

Other High-Protein Foods

- Spirulina (2 tbsp) – 8g protein
- Canned sardines (4 oz) – 28g protein
- Anchovies (4 oz) – 23g protein

Quick Fat Cheat Sheet:

Plant-Based Healthy Fats

- Avocado (1/2 medium) – 12g fat
- Olive oil (1 tbsp, extra virgin) – 14g fat
- Avocado oil (1 tbsp) – 14g fat
- Coconut oil (1 tbsp, unrefined) – 14g fat
- MCT oil (1 tbsp, derived from coconut or palm oil) – 14g fat
- Tahini (2 tbsp, ground sesame seeds) – 16g fat
- Coconut milk (1/2 cup, full-fat canned) – 22g fat

Animal-Based Healthy Fats

- Egg yolks (2 large) – 10g fat
- Salmon (4 oz) – 10g fat
- Sardines (4 oz, canned in olive oil) – 15g fat
- Anchovies (4 oz) – 10g fat
- Beef (4 oz, 85% lean ground beef) – 17g fat
- Lamb (4 oz) – 22g fat
- Duck (4 oz, skin-on) – 20g fat
- Pork (4 oz, pork belly) – 22g fat
- Cheddar cheese (1 oz) – 9g fat
- Mozzarella cheese (1 oz, whole milk) – 7g fat
- Parmesan cheese (1 oz) – 7g fat
- Cottage cheese (1/2 cup, full-fat) – 5g fat

- Greek Yogurt (6 oz, full-fat) – 8g fat
- Butter (1 tbsp, grass-fed) – 11g fat
- Ghee (1 tbsp, clarified butter) – 14g fat

Nuts & Seeds

- Almonds (1 oz, ~23 almonds) – 14g fat
- Walnuts (1 oz, ~14 halves) – 18g fat
- Pecans (1 oz, ~19 halves) – 20g fat
- Macadamia nuts (1 oz, ~10 nuts) – 21g fat
- Cashews (1 oz, ~18 nuts) – 12g fat
- Brazil nuts (1 oz, ~6 nuts) – 19g fat
- Pistachios (1 oz, ~49 nuts) – 13g fat
- Chia seeds (2 tbsp) – 9g fat
- Flax seeds (2 tbsp, ground) – 8g fat
- Hemp seeds (3 tbsp) – 14g fat
- Pumpkin seeds (1 oz, ~85 seeds) – 13g fat
- Sunflower seeds (1 oz, shelled) – 14g fat

Nut & Seed Butters

- Peanut butter (2 tbsp, natural, no sugar added) – 16g fat
- Almond butter (2 tbsp) – 18g fat
- Cashew butter (2 tbsp) – 16g fat
- Sunflower seed butter (2 tbsp) – 16g fat

This method is all about what to ***ADD IN*** to your meals so you feel full, ***fueled***, and balanced.

Chapter 2

E: Exercise Snacks

Welcome to one of our absolute favorite game changers for movement: exercise snacks!

This simple yet powerful habit is part of the foundation of *The Forty Fix* and makes it easy to move consistently without over-complicating your day.

3 walks, 10 minutes each, every day.

These mini bursts of movement are a secret sauce to fat loss. Exercise snacks are backed by science to help with your blood sugar, metabolism, and even hormone balance. Plus, they're easy to squeeze into even the busiest day.

Life can get crazy, and finding time for a full-on workout can feel nearly impossible. Trust us, we've been there. Aimee was juggling becoming a mom of five and managing therapy and doctor appointments for the youngest two, who have higher needs, all while keeping everything afloat with school and sports for the older three.

Erica was in the thick of travel sports and a full-time job, running on empty and trying to squeeze in 5:00 a.m. Orangetheory workouts. But she soon realized those early morning sessions were actually contributing to some of the problems she was facing.

Phew! Tell us exactly when a trip to the gym fits into this life? The truth? You don't have to hit the gym at 5:00 a.m. to be successful.

What if there was a way to work smaller chunks of movement into your day that might actually benefit you in a way a long session gym doesn't?

Enter exercise snacks.

The Magic of Mini-Movements

Why Exercise Snacks?

Exercise snacks are all about those little moments of movement that add up throughout your day. Instead of one long session, think of it as a series of mini workouts that keep you energized and balanced, without the overwhelm.

Often, it seems like our lack of exercise is about time; yes, that's partly true! Let's be real: setting aside an hour for exercise isn't always realistic when you've got a million other things on your plate.

But even more so, it's about our insulin hormone and better blood sugar balance. Because once those are being focused on, *everything* gets easier. Fewer cravings, more energy, fewer crashes, more ease sticking to your plan. And we *all* want that, right?

Three 10-Minute Walks a Day for Better Blood Sugar Balance

Research shows that breaking up long periods of sitting with a few 10-minute walks can really smooth out those post-meal blood sugar glucose spikes.

Even more so, when the walks are strategically timed to be after meals, the effect on lowering glucose spikes is magnified.

In a 2016 study, researchers discovered the following:

> *The iAUC (incremental area under the blood glucose curve) was significantly lower when participants walked after meals compared with on a single daily occasion.*

You can read more about this study here:
https://pubmed.ncbi.nlm.nih.gov/27747394/

How to Make It Work:

- **Morning boost:** Start your day with a brisk 10-minute walk to jumpstart your energy and keep your blood sugar in check.
- **Post-lunch pick-me-up:** A quick 10-minute brisk walk after lunch can help smooth out that post-meal spike.
- **Evening cool-down:** Cap off your day with another 10-minute walk, keeping your metabolism humming and giving your mind a chance to unwind.

Even though a 60-minute walk sounds great in theory, these three shorter walks spaced throughout your day can actually offer even better control over your blood sugar.

Body Squats Every 45 Minutes: A Quick Fix for Your Metabolism

Another little gem? Body squats. Research shows that incorporating simple bodyweight exercises, like squats, every 45 minutes can have a big impact on insulin sensitivity and help reduce those post-meal glucose spikes, much like post-meals walks do. In a 2024 study, researchers highlighted the following:

> *Collectively, short, frequent walking or squatting breaks effectively enhance glycemic control . . . compared to a single bout of walking within prolonged sitting.*

You can check out the study details here:
https://pubmed.ncbi.nlm.nih.gov/38629807/

How to Do It:

- **Set a timer:** Every 45 minutes, pause and do 10–15 squats. It's such a simple way to get your muscles working and keep your blood flowing.

- **Focus on form:** Keep your feet shoulder-width apart and chest lifted, and lower until your thighs are parallel to the floor. A basic squat done right, with this technique, can be super effective.

- **Consistency is key:** These quick squats add up over time, boosting your overall daily activity and countering the negative effects of too much sitting.

When at home during the day and when working (or otherwise unable to walk), ask Alexa to set a timer for 45 minutes. This quick reminder helps you stay on track to move glucose out of the body. As soon as the round of squats is finished, ask Alexa to set a timer for another 45 minutes. This is ideal in an office, at a conference, traveling, or anytime it's not possible to sneak away for a 10-minute walk. It's doable to run off to the bathroom, stretch the legs, or find a private corner to knock out 15 squats quickly before getting back to the meeting.

Exercise Snacks vs. High-Intensity Workouts: A Gentler Touch for Hormonal Balance

We see it too. HIIT classes and Orangetheory are everywhere these days. But here's the thing: for a lot of us (especially those of us fabulous women in our forties), those high-intensity workouts can actually spike cortisol levels, the stress hormone that can lead to stubborn fat storage, and mess with our hormones. Research from a 2008 study reinforces this:

> *Collectively, the cortisol findings support the view that moderate to high-intensity exercise provokes increases in circulating cortisol levels.*

You can read the full article here:
https://pubmed.ncbi.nlm.nih.gov/18787373/

The Perks of Exercise Snacks on Cortisol:

- **Lower stress:** Because these bursts are gentle, they don't send your cortisol levels soaring.

- **Steady energy:** Keeping your body moving in little doses throughout the day helps avoid those energy crashes.

- **Hormonal harmony:** Consistent, moderate movement helps keep cortisol balanced, which is key for overall wellness.

A Simple Routine to Get You Started

The simplest way is to plan ahead! If you're doing 3 walks daily, decide the night before when your walks will be. Write that down in your food journal, which we will talk about in the next chapter. Commit to those times, and then you won't have decision fatigue the day of when you're trying to squeeze them in. After a solid two weeks of 3 walks daily, most of the women we work with find that it becomes routine.

For squat breaks, it can take less planning! Setting a 45-minute timer really helps with keeping up throughout the entire day.

The Power of Exercise Snacks

Exercise snacks are a total powerhouse move. They're simple, research backed, and perfectly tailored for our busy lives. By embracing three 10-minute walks a day or incorporating body squats every 45 minutes, you're actively supporting your blood sugar balance, boosting your metabolism, and keeping your hormones happy, all without the stress of a high-intensity workout or a large time commitment during a full day.

Embrace the power of little bursts of movement and watch as they transform your day, one snack-sized workout at a time.

Real Women, Real Wins

Here's what ladies doing exercise snacks with The 100-50 Method have said:

"I was surprised that incorporating 10-minute walks after meals has increased my steps per day, and I usually end up walking for 15–20 minutes after each meal."
—Dee-Dee N.

"Finding small ways to increase my overall movement is good for the soul! I do traditional weight lifting but realize now

that the little moments of activity are also very important."
—Andrea R. B.

"Love the squats—if I get too busy or am in a hurry and don't have time for a walk, I can always do the squats."
—Jen S.

"Short walks or squats give me a boost of energy."
—Melinda W.

"My favorite way to sneak in movement is doing squats."
—Emily L.

Embrace the power of ***little bursts*** of movement and watch as they ***transform*** your day, one snack-sized workout at a time.

Chapter 3

T: Three Meals a Day

For generations, three meals a day was just how we ate. Breakfast in the morning, a big lunch to refuel midday, and a light dinner to wrap up the day. It was a rhythm and a routine that worked with our body's natural hunger cues.

Somewhere along the way, things changed.

With the rise of the Standard American Diet came a culture of nonstop snacking—granola bars between meetings, a banana and peanut butter during snack time with the kids, handfuls of nuts while making dinner, and those late-night bites in front of the TV.

At some point a shift happened, and we were told that the secret to staying fueled, curbing hunger, boosting metabolism, and keeping our energy up was to eat every three hours. Instead of enjoying three balanced meals, we ended up grazing all day long, thinking it was the way to go.

But here's the thing: science is proving that this shift away from structured meals hasn't done us any favors. Research is now showing that sticking to three well-balanced meals a day is actually better for blood sugar stability, weight management, and even hunger regulation.

Instead of keeping our metabolism "stoked" like we were once told, frequent eating can lead to more insulin spikes, more cravings, and more fat storage. In fact, one groundbreaking study found that eating three meals a day (compared to six) resulted in better weight loss, fewer cravings, and more balanced blood sugar levels.

Here's how it went down. The researchers took twenty-eight people with type 2 diabetes and split them into two groups. Both groups had meals with the same macronutrient composition of fat, protein, and carbohydrates, but with different meal timing, frequency, and distribution over the day.

One group ate three meals a day (think hearty breakfast, solid lunch, light dinner, and no late-night snacking). The other group followed the six-meal approach, with three meals plus three snacks sprinkled throughout the day. Both groups followed their plan for twelve weeks.

The results: after just two weeks, the three-meal-a-day crew had already lost 1.5 kg, while the snacky six-meal group barely budged at 0.3 kg.

Fast-forward to the twelve-week mark, and the differences were even wilder: the three-meal-a-day folks dropped an average of 5.4 kg (that's nearly twelve pounds!), while the six-meal group *gained* 0.3 kg.

And it wasn't just about weight. The three-meal group saw major improvements in blood sugar control. Their HbA1c levels (a measure of blood sugar over time) dropped by 1.2%, while their fasting glucose levels improved more than twice as much as the six-meal group's. Plus, they had significantly fewer cravings, especially for sweets. And here's the coolest part: the study showed eating three meals a day actually helped regulate the genes that control the body's natural rhythms, like sleep, hunger, and metabolism.

The takeaway? Eating three meals a day is about so much more than structure. It's about working *with* your body, not against it. Less hunger, fewer cravings, better blood sugar, and actual weight loss? We call that a major win.

You can read more about this study here:
https://pubmed.ncbi.nlm.nih.gov/31548244/

How Does this Apply to The 100-50 Method?

Eating three balanced meals a day is at the heart and foundation of The 100-50 Method. For women in their forties and beyond, this routine is key to maintaining balanced blood sugar levels and avoiding glucose spikes.

Having three balanced meals a day can help maintain stable blood sugar levels because when you space your meals evenly, you avoid large spikes and dips in blood sugar, which can happen if you skip meals or snack frequently. This consistency helps your body regulate insulin more effectively and supports overall metabolic health. For many, this can lead to better energy levels and a more balanced appetite throughout the day.

Plus, structured meals align with how our bodies naturally burn fat and regulate hunger. That traditional breakfast-lunch-dinner rhythm keeps us full, fuels our metabolism, and prevents the overeating that often follows long fasting periods.

So, What Does This Mean for You?

Knowing that three meals a day is the key to better blood sugar balance, weight loss, and fewer cravings is one thing.

Actually making it happen? That's where the magic of planning comes in.

The reality is, we live in a world that pushes convenience over nourishment, and without a plan, it's easy to fall back into old habits. Setting yourself up for success starts with two powerful tools: food prepping and food journaling. They're game changers when it comes to making three meals a day *work* in your real life.

Food Journaling: Your New Nightly Ritual

For weight loss with The 100-50 Method, a food journal is key! And using it in the most helpful way means writing down all the food you will eat the next day, the **night before**. Food journaling is different from a food log. So often, women tell us they are keeping a food journal, but when we ask about it, we realize it's actually a food log, where you write down what you ate *after* you've had a meal or at the end of the day.

We want you to flip that order around! Now, you're going to use the journal the day *before* to write down your meals for the next day.

Taking a few minutes to plan your meals ahead of time is a total game-changer. It helps you stay intentional, sets you up for success, and lets you make mindful choices before your day even begins. When you're proactive about what you eat, it takes so much pressure off and makes the whole process sustainable.

Why Journal the Night Before?

- **Clarity and commitment:** Writing down your meals ahead gives you a clear roadmap, reducing last-minute, less healthy choices.

- **Balanced nutrition:** Ensures each meal meets your protein and healthy fat targets so your overall daily minimums of 100/50 will be met.

- **Consistency:** Helps maintain regular eating patterns, which are vital for blood sugar stability.

How to Journal Effectively

- **Be specific:** Write down exact portions of protein and healthy fats.

- **Make it routine:** Find a time in the evening when this can be part of your routine. When you do it the same time every day, you will find yourself sticking to it the same way you always brush your teeth before bed or start the dishwasher at the end of the night after tidying up the kitchen.

- **Use an app as an add-on only:** We get it, we all love how apps can make our lives simpler. When it comes to food journaling, though, you don't want to skip the learning process of looking up foods on your own through nutrition labels and writing down the protein and healthy fat yourself. It's totally fine if you decide to also use an app after you write it all down. But as your math teacher would say: show your work first! Take pen to paper the night before and plan out the exact meal you're having with the details of how much protein and healthy fat is in each food. Do this first, and you will quickly become fluent with the amounts to get to your 100/50 minimum goals for the day. We have included a seven-day sample from each of us in the appendix so you can see this tool in action.

Bonus Tip for Food Journaling: Make It a No-Brainer Habit

If you want food journaling to *stick*, the secret sauce is habit stacking, aka pairing it with something you're already doing every night. This simple trick makes it way easier to keep up with, and before you know it, it just becomes second nature.

For Aimee, she loves making it part of her kitchen shut-down routine. After dinner, she washes the dishes, loads the dishwasher, and wipes down the counters, and then before she leaves the kitchen, she sits at the counter and plans out her meals for the next day. The best part? Since she's already *in* the kitchen, if she needs to double-check the protein or healthy fat amounts of something, she can just grab it from the fridge/pantry or do a quick search on her phone. It takes the guesswork out of journaling and makes it feel *seamless*.

For Erica, after running kids to various sports all evening and serving up a second dinner at 8:30 p.m. (some of you might be nodding along), Erica's routine looks a bit different, but the key is it works for her. She makes food journaling part of her nighttime wind-down. After she dives into all things forty-plus skincare (if you know, you know!), she climbs into bed, grabs her journal from the nightstand, and plans out her meals for the next day. Then she emails herself a list of any items she might need to grab at the store. It's easy, and it helps her start the next day feeling more intentional and ready.

The key is to find a routine you *already do* every night and stack your food journaling onto it. When it's built into a habit you're already crushing, it's so much easier to stick with *for good.*

Food Prepping 101: How to Make Three Meals a Day Simple & Stress-Free

Food prepping weekly by having your protein and healthy fats ready to go makes it so much easier to stay consistent and hit your goals. The 100-50 Method is about intentionally choosing foods that support balanced blood sugar, hormone health, and fat loss. And let's be real: when you're hungry and unprepared, it's way too easy to reach for something that'll send your glucose on a rollercoaster.

Prepping your food ahead of time means you're setting yourself up for success, keeping meals simple, and making sure you always have the right foods on hand. Plus, it saves time, reduces stress, and keeps decision fatigue out of the picture.

Top 15 Tips For Food Prepping

1. **Pick your prep day:** Choose a day (Sunday works for most) to plan, shop, and prep your meals for the week.

2. **Start with your proteins:** Cook a batch of chicken, ground turkey, salmon, or steak so you have easy grab-and-go protein options.

3. **Batch cook your veggies:** Roast a tray of broccoli, bell peppers, and zucchini or steam some green beans to pair with meals.

4. **Make a big batch of a staple meal:** Something like a hearty chili, turkey meatballs, or shredded chicken can be repurposed into multiple meals.

5. **Portion it out:** Use glass containers to divide meals ahead of time so they're ready to heat and eat.

6. **Hard-boil some eggs:** This gives you a quick, easy protein source for breakfast or lunch.

7. **Stock your freezer:** Keep frozen veggies, pre-cooked proteins, and emergency meals (like a batch of soup or stew) on hand.

8. **Don't forget healthy fats:** Prep guacamole, portion out nuts, or make a simple dressing with olive oil and lemon juice.

9. **Plan for breakfast:** Chia pudding or pre-made egg muffins can make mornings smoother.

10. **Write it down:** This is where food journaling comes in. Plan your meals the night before so there's no guess-work.

11. **Keep it simple:** You don't need elaborate recipes. Think protein + veggie + healthy fat, and you're good to go.

12. **Have go-to meals on repeat:** Find a few meals you love and rotate them to make things easy.

13. **Prep smart snacks for your kids (not for you!):** If you have little ones, keep their snacks separate so you're not tempted to graze. In our house, we keep their snacks above the fridge so I'm not constantly looking at kid snacks when I open the pantry.

14. **Stick to the basics:** Sometimes preparing *everything* might feel overwhelming. A good place to start is by focusing on the foods that take the longest to cook.

15. **Set yourself up for the week:** Organize your fridge so prepped meals are front and center, making it easier to stay on track.

Real Women, Real Wins

Here is what ladies using The 100-50 Method have said about switching to three meals a day:

> "I love not snacking because (1) I'm not hungry for a snack now and (2) I don't have to figure out what a good/acceptable snack might be! Less planning!!"
> —Sara B.

> "I was eating three main meals and two snacks per day (before this), and now when following the plan and eating veggies,

protein, and then carbs, it keeps me full longer, and I can go four hours without being hungry. Not snacking wasn't hard because I was content from my meals. My mindset challenge was not having coffee before breakfast. This was a huge mindset for me to get over, but I did it and continue to do so."
—Dee-dee N.

"I noticed that I no longer had an afternoon slump when eating three well-balanced meals a day that included 100g protein and 50g healthy fats."
—Stephanie G.

"I'm very mindful of protein now. I just used to be fine with cereal for breakfast because it's fast and easy. You're also hungry in about two hrs. Now, I get 30 to 40 g of protein in the a.m., and it isn't hard to get to lunch."
—Arica H.

"My meals have a ton more protein and fat, and I am satisfied way longer than in the past."
—Emily L.

Instead of keeping our metabolism ***'stoked'*** like we were once told, frequent eating can lead to more insulin spikes, ***more cravings,*** and more fat storage.

CHAPTER 4

H: HORMONES

Out of all the hormones, the one we want to dive really deep into in this chapter is your insulin hormone. Why?

If you're reading this, you're probably wondering why losing weight seems harder and harder as you get older. And you're not alone!

One of the biggest factors involved is insulin, which plays a crucial role in both fat storage and fat burning. It's the hormone that's working behind the scenes in your body every single day, and it could very well be the reason why you feel like your body just isn't cooperating when it comes to shedding those extra pounds.

In order to understand this process so you can fully leverage The 100-50 Method, first it's important to fully understand insulin's purpose in our bodies. This knowledge is what will help you unlock the results with *The Forty Fix*.

What Exactly Is Insulin?

Insulin is a metabolic hormone made by the pancreas. Its primary job is to help control the balance between burning and storing fat in your body. Think of it as your body's traffic controller for energy. When you eat, insulin makes sure glucose (that sweet fuel your body gets from food) is delivered to the cells that need it for energy. So far, so good, right?

Here's how it's *supposed* to work:

1. You eat food (yum).

2. The food turns into glucose (also known as blood sugar).

3. Insulin is released into your bloodstream to carry that glucose to your cells for energy.

Easy enough.

But, like most things in life, it's not always that simple.

The Problem: Insulin Resistance and Its Impact on Weight Loss

Now let's take a deeper look at the problem itself: insulin resistance, which sabotages your body's ability to burn fat and manage weight effectively. You already know that insulin is critical for controlling fat storage and fat burning, but what happens when insulin isn't working properly? That's when things get tricky.

What Happens When Insulin Spikes Too Often?

Here's the problem in simple terms: when insulin is repeatedly elevated, your body stops responding to it the way it should.

This is known as *insulin resistance*. Essentially, your cells begin to ignore insulin's signals to absorb glucose (sugar) from the bloodstream.

The result? Your body ends up circulating higher levels of insulin in an attempt to get glucose into your cells, but because your cells are resistant, it doesn't work as effectively.

This creates a ripple effect, and it's not pretty. Let's break down the consequences:

1. **Fat burning stops:** When insulin is elevated, your body is stuck in "storage mode." Instead of burning

stored fat for energy, your body is focused on dealing with the glucose in your bloodstream. Insulin acts as a fat blocker, preventing the breakdown of fat tissue to be used as energy. Essentially, insulin stops your body from accessing its fat stores, forcing it to hold onto that extra fat instead of burning it.

2. **More fat storage:** Not only does your body stop burning fat, but it starts to store more. Why? Because when insulin is high, it signals your body to store energy (in the form of fat) rather than using it. This is why people with insulin resistance often struggle with weight gain, especially around the belly area. The excess insulin causes your body to store even more fat, further compounding the problem.

3. **Increased hunger and cravings:** High insulin levels make it harder for your body to regulate hunger, which is why you might feel like you're constantly craving sugar, carbs, or junk food. Insulin resistance doesn't just affect your metabolism; it also impacts your brain's hunger signals. As your body becomes resistant to insulin, it struggles to maintain stable blood sugar levels, leading to those all-too-familiar sugar cravings. This causes an endless cycle where you eat more carbs and

sugar, causing even higher insulin levels, which only worsens the resistance.

4. **Vicious cycle of weight gain and insulin resistance:** The problem with insulin resistance is that it creates a vicious cycle. High insulin levels cause fat storage, which leads to more fat, which leads to more insulin resistance. As your fat stores increase, your body becomes less sensitive to insulin, and your cells become more resistant, creating an even bigger challenge when trying to lose weight. This is why it can feel like you're doing everything right (eating healthily, exercising, and sleeping well) but still not seeing results.

Why Does This Happen?

As we age, a lot of things can start shifting in our bodies, and guess what? One of them is how sensitive we are to insulin. That means it gets harder for your body to use glucose the way it should. It can feel like your metabolism is slowing down in all the wrong ways.

So what's behind those insulin spikes that are making weight loss feel like an uphill battle? Here's what could be causing it:

1. A Decrease in Estrogen (Hello, Perimenopause and Menopause)

Estrogen plays a key role in regulating insulin sensitivity. As you age and go through menopause, your estrogen levels drop, which can cause your body to become more resistant to insulin. Translation? Your body has a harder time using insulin properly, making it easier for those extra pounds to stick around.

2. Poor Sleep

You've probably heard it before: sleep is critical for your health. But here's why it's especially important for controlling insulin: when you don't get enough sleep, your insulin sensitivity takes a hit. This means your body isn't able to use insulin as efficiently, and those pesky fat-storing hormones can run wild.

3. Stress

Stress has a sneaky way of affecting your insulin levels. When you're stressed, your body releases cortisol (the "stress hormone"), which can spike your blood sugar and lead to higher insulin levels. Over time, this can contribute to insulin resistance and fat storage.

4. Snacking Often

Constantly snacking throughout the day can lead to frequent insulin spikes. Every time you eat, insulin is released to handle the glucose from your food. If you're constantly eating, you're constantly spiking insulin. This doesn't give your body enough time to reset and burn fat effectively.

5. Eating Too Many Refined Carbs

Carbohydrates are a major source of glucose (blood sugar), so if you're eating a high-carb/processed food diet, you're likely spiking your insulin levels frequently. When insulin is consistently high, it can lead to insulin resistance and difficulty losing weight.

6. Lack of Muscle

Muscle tissue helps increase your body's insulin sensitivity. The more muscle you have, the more efficient your body is at using insulin. If you're not getting enough exercise or strength training, your insulin sensitivity may decline.

7. Excess Weight, Especially Belly Fat

Carrying extra weight, particularly around your abdomen, can negatively affect insulin sensitivity. Fat cells in your belly can release hormones that interfere with insulin's ability to do its job.

The more belly fat you carry, the harder it is for your body to use insulin effectively.

The Surprising Impact on Fat Storage

One of the most frustrating aspects of insulin resistance is how it affects your fat distribution, especially around your belly and bra line bulge, as we call it. This "abdominal fat" isn't just a concern for fitting into your clothes; it's also a metabolic one. Belly fat, or visceral fat, is the fat that wraps around your internal organs, and it's particularly resistant to fat-burning processes.

This kind of fat produces inflammatory chemicals and hormones that make it even harder for your body to burn fat. In fact, the more belly fat you have, the more your body releases substances that exacerbate insulin resistance, leading to even higher insulin levels. This makes it a stubborn, hard-to-shift kind of fat.

Why You Feel Like You're Gaining Weight Out of Nowhere

One of the most frustrating things about insulin resistance is that it often feels like you're gaining weight out of nowhere. You might not have changed your diet or exercise habits, but the scale keeps creeping up. This can feel incredibly disheartening and confusing, especially if you're doing everything "right." Unfortunately, this is a very common experience for those dealing with insulin resistance.

Your body is no longer responding to insulin the way it used to, and as a result, your metabolism slows down. Even if you're still eating the same foods or working out like you used to, your body's ability to burn calories effectively decreases. It's like your body's metabolism is stuck in first gear, while your insulin levels keep revving higher and higher.

Now that we understand how insulin resistance can impact fat storage and weight loss, let's get into the practical, actionable tips that will help you boost insulin sensitivity and break the cycle. These steps aren't just about weight loss; they're about improving your overall metabolic health and feeling better in your body.

Knowing whether your insulin or blood sugar levels are off is essential for managing your overall health, especially if you're concerned about insulin resistance or metabolic issues. The following section gives some signs, symptoms, and tests to help you determine if your insulin or blood sugar levels might be out of balance.

Signs That Your Insulin or Blood Sugar Levels Could Be Off

We call these red flags, signs that your insulin or blood sugar levels could be out of balance. These clues are your body's way of saying, "Hey, something's not quite right here!" So if you're experiencing any of these, it might be time to tune in and take action. Here are the big signs that things could be off, and what to look for:

1. **Frequent Hunger and Cravings for Sugar or Carbs**
    - When your insulin levels are elevated and your body becomes resistant to insulin, you may experience persistent hunger. Your body may crave high-carb or sugary foods as it seeks a quick source of energy.
    - **Why this happens:** Insulin resistance can prevent your cells from receiving glucose, leaving you feeling hungry even though your blood sugar may actually be high.
2. **Fatigue or Feeling Drained**
    - Sudden fatigue after eating, especially after consuming a meal high in carbs, is a common sign of blood sugar imbalances.
    - **Why this happens:** When insulin isn't functioning properly, glucose can't enter your cells to provide energy, leaving you feeling sluggish or tired.

3. **Increased Thirst or Frequent Urination**

    - High blood sugar levels often lead to dehydration because your body tries to get rid of excess glucose through urine. This results in increased thirst and frequent trips to the bathroom.

    - **Why this happens:** When blood sugar levels rise, the kidneys work overtime to filter out excess glucose, causing fluid loss.

4. **Unexplained Weight Gain (Especially Around the Belly)**

    - Insulin is a fat-storage hormone. When your body becomes insulin resistant, it may lead to weight gain, particularly around the abdomen. This is because the body is storing excess glucose as fat.

    - **Why this happens:** The more insulin your body produces to compensate for its resistance, the more it encourages fat storage.

5. **Difficulty Losing Weight**

    - If you're eating well and exercising but find it hard to shed pounds, it could be a sign of insulin resistance.

The body's inability to properly regulate insulin can make weight loss difficult, even with a healthy diet and exercise.

- **Why this happens:** Insulin resistance slows down fat-burning processes, making it harder for your body to tap into stored fat for energy.

6. **Brain Fog or Trouble Concentrating**

    - Consistently elevated blood sugar levels can interfere with cognitive function. This can lead to feelings of brain fog, difficulty focusing, or trouble remembering things.

    - **Why this happens:** Blood sugar imbalances affect brain chemistry, which can impair mental clarity and focus.

7. **Dark Skin Patches (Acanthosis Nigricans)**

    - One of the more visible signs of insulin resistance is the development of dark, velvety skin patches, usually in areas like the neck, armpits, or groin.

    - **Why this happens:** Acanthosis nigricans occurs due to the overproduction of insulin, which stimulates skin cells to grow rapidly, creating these dark patches.

8. **Frequent Infections or Slow-Healing Wounds**

    - Elevated blood sugar levels can weaken your immune system, making it harder for your body to fight infections. Wounds may take longer to heal as well.

    - **Why this happens:** High blood sugar levels can impair the immune system's ability to respond to infections and can hinder wound healing due to poor circulation.

When to Seek Medical Help

If you experience any combination of the signs listed above, especially if they persist for an extended period, it's important to consult with your doctor. Insulin resistance and high blood sugar are often early warning signs of type 2 diabetes and can lead to other serious health issues, including cardiovascular disease.

Your Doctor May Order:

- **Fasting insulin test** to assess insulin resistance

- **Thyroid function test** (as thyroid imbalances can influence insulin sensitivity)
- **Lipid profile** to check cholesterol levels (since high insulin levels often correlate with high cholesterol)

Your Doctor May Also Look into Blood Sugar Levels Being Off:

1. **Fasting Blood Sugar Test**
    - This is one of the simplest and most common tests. It measures your blood sugar after an overnight fast (usually eight to twelve hours without food).
    - **Normal range:** Less than 100 mg/dL
    - **Pre-diabetes:** 100-125 mg/dL
    - **Diabetes:** 126 mg/dL or higher
2. **Oral Glucose Tolerance Test (OGTT)**
    - In this test, you'll drink a sugary solution, and your blood sugar will be measured at intervals afterward to see how your body handles the glucose. It's often used to diagnose gestational diabetes and can also help identify insulin resistance or prediabetes.

- **Normal range:** Less than 140 mg/dL at two hours
- **Pre-Diabetes:** 140-199 mg/dL at two hours
- **Diabetes:** 200 mg/dL or higher at two hours

3. **Hemoglobin A1c Test**
    - The A1c test measures your average blood sugar levels over the past two to three months. This test is useful for diagnosing diabetes and monitoring long-term blood sugar control.
    - **Normal range:** Below 5.7%
    - **Pre-diabetes:** 5.7%–6.4%
    - **Diabetes:** 6.5% or higher
4. **Insulin Sensitivity or Resistance Test**
    - An insulin resistance test measures the level of insulin in your blood after a glucose load or in response to a fasting state. Higher levels of insulin in the blood after fasting or consuming glucose indicate insulin resistance.
    - **Home testing:** You can also use a home insulin resistance calculator that combines your blood sugar

and insulin levels to estimate your insulin sensitivity.

5. **Continuous Glucose Monitor (CGM)**

   - A CGM is a small device that you wear on your skin that continuously measures your blood glucose levels throughout the day. It can give you real-time data on how your blood sugar fluctuates in response to food, exercise, and stress.

   - **Why it helps:** By seeing the fluctuations in blood sugar, you can better understand how different foods and habits impact your insulin and blood sugar levels.

6. **C-Peptide Test**

   - This test measures the level of C-peptide in the blood, which is released when insulin is produced. High levels of C-peptide can indicate that your body is producing more insulin to overcome insulin resistance.

   - **Why it helps:** This can help identify if the body is overproducing insulin as a response to insulin resistance.

Tips for Boosting Insulin Sensitivity

Here's the good news: there's so much you can do to help your body become more sensitive to insulin and break free from that endless cycle of fat storage.

You're not stuck, and you definitely don't have to just "accept" it. The power is in your hands!

So, let's talk about some simple, actionable steps you can start taking today to get your body back on track.

1. Balance Your Meals with Protein & Healthy Fats (The 100-50 Method)

Instead of relying on quick snacks or high-carb meals that spike your insulin, focus on eating balanced meals that help keep your blood sugar steady. When your blood sugar stays stable, insulin doesn't need to spike as much.

- **Protein:** Include lean proteins like chicken, turkey, tofu, eggs, and fish. Protein helps balance blood sugar levels and keeps you feeling full longer.

- **Healthy fats:** Avocados, olive oil, nuts, seeds, and fatty fish (like salmon) are great sources of healthy fats that help regulate insulin and support fat burning.

- **Fiber:** Non-starchy vegetables (like leafy greens, broccoli, and cauliflower), whole grains (like quinoa), and legumes (beans, lentils) are high in fiber, which helps slow the digestion of carbohydrates and keeps insulin levels stable.

2. Incorporate Exercise Snacks

As we discussed in chapter 2, "Exercise Snacks," short, brisk walks or body squats throughout the day have a big impact on insulin sensitivity. When strategically planned for after meals, exercise snacks help reduce those post-meal glucose spikes.

3. Prioritize Sleep for Better Insulin Sensitivity

Poor sleep can contribute to insulin resistance, so getting quality rest is essential for balancing your hormones and metabolism. Aim for seven to nine hours of uninterrupted sleep each night.

- **Create a sleep routine:** Set a consistent bedtime and wake-up time to regulate your circadian rhythm.

- **Avoid electronics before bed:** The blue light from screens can interfere with melatonin production, making it harder for you to fall asleep.

- **Create a relaxing sleep environment:** Keep your bedroom cool, dark, and quiet, and use calming activities (like reading or meditation) before bed.

4. Support Your Gut Health

Emerging research shows that gut health plays a crucial role in insulin sensitivity. A healthy gut microbiome can help regulate blood sugar levels and reduce inflammation in the body.

- **Eat fermented foods:** Sauerkraut, kimchi, yogurt (with no added sugar), and kefir are great for boosting gut health.

- **Increase fiber:** Foods high in fiber, such as beans, lentils, whole grains, and vegetables, help promote a healthy gut and support stable blood sugar.

5. Cut Back on Refined Carbs and Sugar

Refined carbs and sugars cause rapid spikes in blood glucose and insulin levels. By cutting back on these foods, you can improve your insulin sensitivity and reduce fat storage.

- **Avoid sugary beverages:** Soda, sweetened coffee drinks, and fruit juices can cause rapid insulin spikes. Opt for water, herbal tea, or unsweetened coffee instead.

- **Limit processed carbs:** Skip foods like white bread, pastries, and processed snacks. Instead, choose whole grains like brown rice, quinoa, or sweet potatoes.

- **Choose low-glycemic foods:** Foods with a lower glycemic index (GI) help prevent sharp rises in blood sugar. Think non-starchy veggies, legumes, and whole fruits (like berries and apples).

6. Increase Your Omega-3 Fatty Acids

Omega-3 fatty acids are anti-inflammatory and can help reduce insulin resistance. They're also essential for overall heart and metabolic health.

- **Eat fatty fish:** Salmon, mackerel, sardines, and other fatty fish are excellent sources of omega-3s.

- **Plant-based omega-3s:** Walnuts, chia seeds, flaxseeds, and hemp seeds also provide omega-3s if you prefer plant-based sources.

7. Consider Supplements for Insulin Sensitivity (with Medical Approval)

Certain supplements may support insulin sensitivity, but always consult with your healthcare provider before adding anything new to your routine.

- **Magnesium:** This mineral is important for insulin

function. Foods rich in magnesium include leafy greens, nuts, seeds, and whole grains.

- **Berberine:** This plant extract has been shown to help improve insulin sensitivity
- **Cinnamon:** Cinnamon has been linked to improved blood sugar regulation. Try adding it to smoothies, oatmeal, or coffee.

The Role of Hormones Beyond Insulin

While insulin might be the headline act when it comes to metabolic regulation, it's not the only hormone in the show. There are a few other behind-the-scenes players that can impact how well your body responds to insulin and how it handles fat storage. These hormones have a big role in how your body balances everything, so let's dive into the ones you should know about:

Leptin: Known as the "satiety hormone," leptin helps regulate appetite and fat storage. However, in insulin resistance, leptin's effectiveness decreases (known as *leptin resistance*), leading to increased hunger and difficulty losing weight.

- **Action tip:** Focus on eating whole, nutrient-dense meals to help balance leptin levels. Also, avoid overeating processed foods that can exacerbate leptin resistance.

Ghrelin: Often referred to as the "hunger hormone," ghrelin stimulates appetite and food intake. When insulin resistance is present, ghrelin levels can become imbalanced, leading to increased cravings for high-carb or high-sugar foods.

- **Action tip:** Aim to keep your meals high in protein and fiber to keep ghrelin levels in check, ensuring you're not constantly fighting hunger and cravings.

Thyroid hormones: Thyroid imbalances (such as hypothyroidism) can slow down metabolism, making it harder to burn fat and regulate insulin. Hypothyroidism often coincides with insulin resistance, which further complicates weight management.

- **Action tip:** Get your thyroid function tested regularly, especially if you're experiencing unexplained weight gain or fatigue. Consider a diet rich in iodine (found in seaweed) and selenium (found in Brazil nuts) to support thyroid health.

Growth hormone: This hormone, which peaks during childhood and adolescence, plays a role in fat metabolism. As we age, growth hormone levels decline, which can contribute to the accumulation of fat, especially belly fat.

- **Action tip:** Intermittent fasting and high-intensity exercise have been shown to boost growth hormone levels naturally. Adding strength training can help preserve lean muscle mass, which helps maintain healthy insulin levels.

Common Mistakes and Pitfalls That You'll Avoid with The 100-50 Method

Managing insulin resistance and balancing blood sugar can feel like navigating a maze, right? You're trying to do all the right things, but it's easy to trip up along the way, which can totally slow your progress or even make things worse.

This is where The 100-50 Method has you covered. Here are some of the most common slip-ups people make when it comes to managing insulin resistance, plus simple, actionable tips to help you steer clear of them. Trust us, these tweaks can make a huge difference!

1. Relying Too Much on "Low-Carb" Diets without Understanding the Quality of Carbs

Mistake: Many people turn to low-carb or ketogenic diets in an effort to control insulin levels, thinking that cutting carbs is the only solution. While reducing carbohydrates can be beneficial for some, focusing on the quality of carbs is just as important as quantity.

- **Pitfall:** Not all carbs are created equal. Cutting out all carbohydrates (especially healthy ones like fruits, vegetables, and whole grains) can lead to nutrient deficiencies. Many low-carb diets also promote processed and unhealthy fats, which can worsen inflammation and insulin resistance.

- **Solution:** With The 100-50 Method, instead of completely eliminating carbs, you focus on low-glycemic, high-fiber carbohydrates. These slow down the release of glucose into the bloodstream and improve insulin sensitivity. Think whole grains (quinoa), vegetables (leafy greens, cauliflower), and fruits (berries, apples).

2. Not Prioritizing Protein and Fiber in Meals

Mistake: A common error is focusing primarily on carbs or fats while neglecting the importance of protein and fiber in balancing blood sugar levels. Both protein and fiber play critical roles in slowing down the absorption of sugar and maintaining stable blood sugar levels.

- **Pitfall:** Meals that are too high in carbs and fats, without enough protein or fiber, can cause blood sugar spikes and contribute to insulin resistance over time.

- **Solution:** With The 100-50 Method, the goal is to include protein (like chicken, turkey, fish, tofu, or beans) and fiber-rich foods (like leafy greens, broccoli, and chia seeds) in every meal. This helps slow the digestion of carbohydrates, preventing rapid spikes in blood sugar.

3. Overdoing "Healthy" Snacks and Treats

Mistake: Healthy snacks like granola bars, smoothies, and fruit can still lead to insulin spikes if consumed in excess. Even though these foods are marketed as "healthier," they may contain hidden sugars, unhealthy fats, or refined carbohydrates that negatively impact blood sugar control.

- **Pitfall:** Over-consuming even healthy snacks, such as fruit or granola, can lead to higher insulin levels and disrupt blood sugar balance. People also often snack mindlessly, leading to extra calorie intake that can contribute to weight gain.

- **Solution:** With The 100-50 Method, stick to three meals a day to avoid snacking. Focus on whole foods and try to avoid pre-packaged items or those with added sugar. If you're eating fruit, opt for low-glycemic fruits like berries, try pairing them with a protein or fat to help stabilize blood sugar, and put fruit at the end of the meal.

4. Focusing Too Much on Cardio and Not Enough on Walking

Mistake: Many people believe that cardio exercises (like running or cycling) are the best way to manage blood sugar and insulin resistance. While cardio is beneficial, it's not the most efficient way to increase insulin sensitivity and improve overall metabolic health.

- **Pitfall:** Relying solely on cardio can limit your progress because it doesn't build muscle mass, which is key for improving insulin sensitivity. Additionally, too much cardio without strength training may cause muscle loss, which can negatively affect metabolism.
- **Solution:** Incorporate both aerobic exercises (walking, jogging, swimming) and/or strength training (weight lifting, resistance exercises, bodyweight exercises). Building muscle helps improve insulin sensitivity and supports fat loss. Aim for a balanced routine that includes both types of exercise.

5. Skipping Meals or Fasting for Too Long

Mistake: Some people turn to intermittent fasting or skip meals with the belief that it will lead to quicker weight loss and improved blood sugar regulation. However, skipping meals can lead to low blood sugar (hypoglycemia), which can cause fatigue, dizziness, and irritability, and even worsen insulin resistance over time.

- **Pitfall:** Long periods of fasting or skipping meals can slow your metabolism, increase stress hormones like cortisol, and make your body more prone to insulin resistance. It also increases the risk of overeating later in the day, which can contribute to blood sugar spikes.

- **Solution:** Eating three meals a day with The 100-50 Method will already provide a fasting window from twelve to fourteen hours (dinner to breakfast the next morning). Instead of prolonging a fast by skipping meals, aim for three balanced meals throughout the day to keep blood sugar levels stable.

6. Neglecting Sleep and Stress Management

Mistake: Sleep and stress play significant roles in insulin sensitivity, but many people overlook their impact. Chronic stress and lack of sleep can elevate cortisol, which in turn raises blood sugar and leads to insulin resistance.

- **Pitfall:** Stress, whether physical or emotional, triggers the release of cortisol, which can increase insulin levels and contribute to fat storage, especially around the abdomen. Poor sleep quality also disrupts glucose metabolism, making it harder for your body to regulate blood sugar effectively.

- **Solution:** Prioritize sleep by aiming for seven to nine hours of quality sleep each night. Practice stress management techniques such as mindfulness, meditation, deep breathing exercises, or yoga. Managing both your physical and mental stress can significantly improve insulin sensitivity.

Wrapping It Up

As you can see, insulin is *the* key player when it comes to the tug-of-war between fat storage and fat burning. And as we get older, our bodies can start to lose their sensitivity to it, making it way easier to pack on pounds and harder to shed them. The good news is, with The 100-50 Method and the right strategies in place, you can absolutely turn things around.

Real Women, Real Wins

Here's what a few of the women we've worked with have to say about how The 100-50 Method has improved their blood sugar and insulin balance:

"I did not realize how crucial having balanced blood sugar would be for my mood."
—Emily L.

"I am not tired in the afternoons (3:00) anymore and not craving chips (my biggest downfall)."
—Dee-Dee N.

"I think having a good balance of protein and fat helped my insulin balance because I feel a steady energy now."
—Andrea R. B.

"I am an RN, so I already knew about insulin resistance. I had gestational diabetes for all five of my pregnancies and miscarried twice after being told I was insulin resistant. What I did not know was how insulin resistance increased my fat storage and made it so difficult to lose weight."
—Stephanie G.

Insulin is your body's traffic ***controller*** for energy—deciding whether to ***burn fat*** or store it.

Chapter 5

O: Optimization

By now, you've got the foundation down. You know how powerful The 100-50 Method can be for fueling your body and feeling your best. But what if we could take it up a notch? What if there was a way to fine-tune this method and make it work even harder for you?

That's where optimization comes in. In this chapter, we're going to talk about one way to take this method even further: your GLP-1 hormone. Dialing in on this can help you feel fuller and more balanced and see even better results. It is an effective way to accelerate the transformation you will experience with *The Forty Fix*.

Optimizing The 100-50 Method with GLP-1

Want to know something that gets us *really* excited?

It's the intersection of GLP-1 (that's glucagon-like peptide-1) hormones and The 100-50 Method to optimize your weight loss.

This chapter is going to unpack some of the latest science, break down how GLP-1 plays into weight loss and overall wellness, and teach you how to optimize your nutrition with The 100-50 Method by focusing on boosting this hormone.

The chatter around GLP-1, especially in the form of weight loss shots like Ozempic, Wegovy, and Trulicity, can be overwhelming. But let's not forget that whether you're opting for nature's version (through food, lifestyle, and gut health optimization) or going with the peptide-assisted route (or doing both!), optimizing your approach is *key* to seeing real, sustainable results.

Before we dive in, one last quick note: The 100-50 Method is for *everyone.*

If you're here for a food-and-lifestyle-based approach to managing weight, balancing hormones, and supporting GLP-1 levels, you're in exactly the right place. This method was built around the power of real food, daily habits, and consistency.

And if you're here because you're using GLP-1 medication *and* looking to build real, sustainable habits that protect your muscle, balance your meals, and support long-term health? We see you, we celebrate you, and we're so glad you're here.

Our community includes women following both paths. The beauty of The 100-50 Method is the flexibility; it's designed to meet you exactly where you are.

In this chapter, we'll explore both approaches. Feel free to skip ahead if a particular section doesn't apply to you.

The Basics

Let's kick things off with the basics: GLP-1 is a hormone that's actually made in your gut. Yep, you heard that right—in your gut! And, no, it's not just about digestion. This hormone does some heavy lifting when it comes to keeping your metabolism on track and regulating your blood sugar.

Here's how GLP-1 works in your body:

1. **Regulates blood sugar:** GLP-1 helps keep blood sugar levels balanced, preventing the glucose spikes and crashes that leave you feeling like you're on an exhaustion roller coaster. It slows gastric emptying, meaning your stomach takes longer to empty after eating. This helps you feel full longer and gives your body more time to absorb nutrients.

2. **Appetite control:** One of the big players in weight loss, GLP-1 suppresses appetite. It sends signals to your brain telling you you're full. It's like having a natural, built-in off switch for cravings.

3. **Fat metabolism:** Beyond just controlling hunger, GLP-1 has been shown to influence fat metabolism (the process of the digestion, absorption, synthesis, and decomposition of human lipids). If you've ever felt like your body just refuses to burn fat no matter what you do, GLP-1 could be part of solving the puzzle.

The Women's Factor: Losing GLP-1?

For many women, especially as they age or go through significant hormonal changes (think pregnancy, menopause), the natural production of GLP-1 can start to drop. And that's a tough pill to swallow, especially if you're trying to maintain a healthy weight or balance your blood sugar.

Here's why this happens: estrogen, the primary female hormone, influences GLP-1 secretion. As estrogen levels fluctuate, especially during perimenopause or menopause, the body's ability to produce GLP-1 naturally can decrease. This can lead to weight gain, increased cravings, and difficulty managing blood sugar levels.

- **Hormonal fluctuations:** Women are more sensitive to hormonal fluctuations, which can affect appetite and metabolism. By optimizing GLP-1 production through food and lifestyle, women can combat some of the negative effects of hormone imbalances that come with aging, menstruation, and other life stages.

- **Sustainable weight loss:** Using food and lifestyle to optimize your GLP-1 levels creates a sustainable, long-term approach that helps you manage your weight. Balanced eating, gut health, exercise, and stress management can all help support your GLP-1.

Leaning into Your GLP-1 Levels Naturally: A Holistic Approach for Women

Boosting your GLP-1 levels starts with what you put in your body, how you treat your gut, the way you move, and the lifestyle choices you make. It's all about setting yourself up for success by feeding your body the right foods, prioritizing gut health, staying active, and managing stress. When you do all this, you're helping your body naturally ramp up its GLP-1 production, which means better metabolism, more control over hunger, and (as you might have guessed already) fat loss.

It's about working *with* your body, not against it. You've got the tools to make this happen, and when you're intentional about your approach, you'll start seeing those incredible changes in the way your body responds.

Let's break this down into the actionable steps you can take:

1. Eat to Stimulate GLP-1 Naturally:

The food you eat plays a huge role in naturally boosting GLP-1 production. It's all about choosing nutrient-dense foods that support hormone regulation and gut health. Here's how:

- **Healthy fats:** Healthy fats are crucial for hormone production, including GLP-1. Aim for about 50 g of healthy fat daily, focusing on monounsaturated fats and omega-3 fatty acids. Avocados, olive oil, coconut oil, nuts, and seeds are fantastic sources. These fats also help maintain blood sugar levels, which directly supports GLP-1's function in appetite regulation and fat metabolism.

- **Protein:** Protein is key to stimulating GLP-1 release. Aim for around 100g of protein minimum per day, spread throughout your meals. Protein triggers the release of GLP-1 and helps build lean muscle, which in turn supports fat burning. Good sources include meats (chicken, turkey), eggs, fatty fish (salmon, sardines), tofu, tempeh, and legumes like lentils and chickpeas.

- **Fiber-rich foods:** High-fiber foods are essential for gut health and indirectly support GLP-1 production. Fiber feeds your good gut bacteria, which helps maintain a healthy microbiome that produces more GLP-1. Focus on vegetables, fruits, whole grains, beans, and legumes. The more fiber you eat, the better your gut functions and the better GLP-1 gets to work!

- **Fermented foods:** Probiotics and prebiotics are the backbone of a healthy gut, which is directly linked to GLP-1 production. Fermented foods like sauerkraut, kimchi, kefir, and yogurt help populate your gut with beneficial bacteria that can enhance GLP-1 secretion. Eating a variety of fermented foods supports a diverse gut microbiome, which is essential for optimal hormone production and metabolism.

- **Spices and herbs:** Certain herbs and spices also support your gut health and metabolism. Turmeric, ginger, and cinnamon are known to have anti-inflammatory properties and can help regulate blood sugar, indirectly boosting GLP-1. Adding these to your meals can provide an extra metabolic boost!

Does all of this sound familiar? So much of what we discussed with The 100-50 Method in previous chapters can also help with naturally boosting your GLP-1 levels.

2. Gut Health: The Key to GLP-1 Production

Here is something that might surprise you: your gut microbiome is actually one of the *biggest players* in the GLP-1 game. When your gut bacteria are healthy and balanced, they help your body produce more GLP-1, which is like the secret sauce for keeping your appetite in check and getting your metabolism firing on all cylinders.

The flip side of that, though, is that if your gut is out of whack, it can totally mess with GLP-1 release. When that happens, you might find yourself dealing with more hunger, those *insane* cravings, and trouble managing your weight. This is why your gut health is a BIG deal when it comes to GLP-1. Take care of it, and you're setting yourself up for success.

How to optimize your gut health:

- **Prebiotics:** Prebiotics are the fiber-based foods that feed the good bacteria in your gut. Think of prebiotics as the fuel that powers the healthy microbes. These can be found in foods like garlic, onions, asparagus, bananas, and leeks. Including these in your meals regularly is a great way to support a thriving gut microbiome.

- **Probiotics:** As mentioned, fermented foods are a great source of probiotics. But you can also incorporate probiotic supplements into your routine if needed. Probiotics help restore and maintain the balance of healthy bacteria in your gut, which is essential for natural GLP-1 production.

- **Avoid gut disruptors:** Certain foods and environmental factors can negatively affect your gut. Processed foods, excess sugar, artificial sweeteners, and chronic stress can all harm the delicate balance of your gut microbiome. Reducing or eliminating these disruptors from your diet can give your gut the best chance to thrive and support GLP-1 production.

Peptide-Based Weight Loss: The GLP-1 Revolution

Let's dive into something that's fascinating: peptide therapy. GLP-1 therapies are peptides that mimic your body's natural GLP-1 production.

Here's the thing about peptides: they're like little messengers in your body, telling your cells exactly what to do. With GLP-1, for example, this leads to a more balanced appetite, better fat burning, and an overall healthier metabolism.

GLP-1 agonists, like Ozempic, are essentially a synthetic version of GLP-1, designed to mimic the natural hormone's effects. When you inject it, it goes straight to work, helping regulate blood sugar, curb cravings, and promote fat burning.

Here's where things get really interesting. Micro-dosing GLP-1 therapy is gaining traction in the biohacking world, especially among functional medicine doctors and naturopathic practitioners. Instead of using standard doses, micro-dosing involves taking much smaller amounts of GLP-1 agonists. These low doses help maintain steady levels in the body, delivering the metabolic benefits without the common side effects like nausea or stomach upset that can come with higher doses. Research shows that micro-dosing can significantly improve insulin sensitivity and reduce inflammation, making it a powerful tool for metabolic health.

Disclaimer: The information provided in this content is for educational and informational purposes only and is not intended as medical advice. GLP-1 therapies, including peptide-based treatments, should be used under the supervision of a qualified healthcare provider. Always consult with your physician or a licensed medical professional before starting, stopping, or changing any medication, supplement, or treatment plan. Individual results may vary, and what works for one person may not be appropriate for another.

The 100-50 Method: A Nutrient-Dense Approach

Why GLP-1 Therapy Works with The 100-50 Method (And How You Can Optimize It)

Whether you go the natural route or use peptides (or both!), the real key is optimization.

1. **Combine GLP-1 with the right nutrition:** As mentioned earlier, hitting that 100/50 (100g of protein and 50g of healthy fat) works hand in hand with GLP-1 regulation. These nutrients fuel your body in a way that supports GLP-1 production, while also helping you maintain muscle mass and keeping your hormones balanced.

2. **Gut health is your secret weapon:** Here's where things get *really* interesting. GLP-1 isn't just about the hormone itself; it's heavily influenced by your gut microbiome. An imbalanced gut can wreak havoc on GLP-1 levels, which is why probiotics, prebi-

otics, and fiber-rich foods are a must. When your gut is healthy, GLP-1 production soars, and you'll feel fuller for longer. It's like a natural booster shot for your metabolism!

3. **Lifestyle & movement matter:** Exercise (particularly strength training and cardio) increases GLP-1 secretion naturally. So whether you're on peptides or optimizing through food, making movement a consistent part of your routine can amplify the effects of GLP-1 on your metabolism. The more active you are, the more GLP-1 your body produces, which, in turn, helps with appetite control and fat burning.

This hormone is the key to unlocking a balanced, efficient metabolism and helping you keep cravings in check. And gut health is a HUGE piece of the puzzle. When you focus on nourishing your gut, you're setting your body up to naturally boost GLP-1 production. Add in The 100-50 Method, and you've got a game plan that will supercharge your results.

When you combine all of this (peptides, gut health, The 100-50 Method), you're creating the perfect environment for GLP-1 to thrive. And that means you're on the fast track to achieving results. So whether you're looking to transform your metabolism, keep your hunger in check, or kick-start fat loss, these tools and strategies are your key to success. It's about smart, sustainable choices that work *with* your body, not against it.

Real Women, Real Wins

Here are just a few words from women who have optimized their GLP with The 100-50 Method:

> "I've been adding in fermented foods to the beginning of my meal, and it's become part of my natural routine. I add chia seeds to a lot of my foods, too, for the GLP-1 boost, and I've noticed I really do stay fuller longer."
> —Sarah B.

> "A few months ago, I decided to try GLP-1 medication after seeing the benefits in friends my age. But I was worried about losing muscle in the process. My friend shared The 100-50 Method Instagram with me, and that changed everything: 100 grams of protein a day, short daily walks, and intentional habits to maintain muscle while on the medication. It took effort to hit those protein goals, but it's been worth it. I've lost twenty pounds and kept my muscle, and I'm building new habits."
> —Jenn B.

When you focus on ***nourishing*** your gut, you're setting your body up to ***naturally boost*** GLP-1 production. Add in The 100-50 Method, and you've got a game plan that will s***upercharge your results.***

Chapter 6

D: Daily

Habits create results.

Food journaling is a habit. Hitting your 100/50 goal each day is a habit. Doing three walks a day is a habit. Eating all your nourishment during three meals a day is a habit.

The things we've covered in the previous chapters are all about creating these little habits that add up to big results. The best way to make them stick? Do them daily.

In his book *Atomic Habits*, James Clear emphasizes that small, consistent actions lead to significant improvements over time. "Habits are the compound interest of self-improvement," he states, highlighting how daily consistency leads to remarkable results.

It's those small, daily habits that truly shape our journey. Think of it as a snowball effect; each tiny action adds up, creating a momentum that can lead to incredible transformation.

When it comes to doing these habits daily, we have two pro tips for you—track and stack.

Habit Tracking

One thing that is helpful is to focus on keeping a streak. Whether it's sticking to three balanced meals a day, getting in your daily walks, or consistently hitting 100 grams of protein and 50 grams of healthy fats, the goal of keeping a streak going builds momentum.

For example, when we first got started with making sure we were hitting 100/50 daily, we each put a paper calendar (the kind with a box for each day) in a cabinet in the kitchen. At the end of each day, we were so excited to give ourselves a checkmark and text each other to celebrate knocking it out. Once we built a streak (even if it was just a few days), we didn't want it to end. No matter what life threw at us, we weren't about to break that streak. We stayed focused on hitting 100/50 every single day, just for that little checkmark. It was all about keeping the momentum going.

The goal is to create a streak of checkmarks, which builds motivation to keep going. It's a simple yet powerful visual reminder of your progress!

Start with one streak and focus on maintaining it. Once it becomes second nature, like it's part of who you are, add another layer. This approach not only builds consistency but also ensures sustainable progress.

Habit Stacking

Once you've built a foundation with tracking, it's time to bring in the second pro tip: stacking. Habit stacking is a concept coined by James Clear in *Atomic Habits*, and it's exactly what it sounds like—stacking a new habit onto one that's already solid in your routine. It's about using what's already working as the anchor for something new you want to add in.

Why does this matter? Because it's much easier to remember and implement a new behavior when it's tied to something you're already doing. It creates rhythm and flow instead of decision fatigue.

Here's a simple example. Let's say you walk your kids to the bus stop every morning. That's your anchor. You could stack a new habit on top of it by doing a brisk ten-minute walk around the neighborhood once they get on the bus. This turns what could be an "I'll do it later" task into an automatic part of your routine.

Or maybe after you brush your teeth at night, you have a streak calendar on the inside of your bathroom cabinet to do a quick check-in: "Did I nourish myself well today with three meals?" Check! That is when you stack on your daily tracking.

These little stacks build an intentional rhythm into your day.

Habit stacking works best when it's specific and tied to a clear cue. Instead of vaguely deciding you'll "walk more," you anchor it to something concrete: "After I finish lunch, I'll take a ten-minute walk." That becomes your new pattern, and walks aren't random anymore, they're part of your daily loop. You can even build a habit chain where several behaviors become stacked together. It's like setting up dominoes that fall in your favor every single day.

What makes this so effective is that it removes the guesswork. You're not relying on willpower or motivation, which, let's be honest, can be MIA some days. Instead, you're relying on systems. Stacking your habits means they start running in the background, like a well-oiled machine. This is how you become the kind of person who just naturally walks, naturally hits 100/50, naturally plans meals. It's not because you're trying harder; it's because your day is built to support you.

As you get more comfortable, you can start to layer more stacks into your day. But the magic is in keeping it simple and doable. One stack at a time. One loop that leads to the next. Over time, these small, stacked actions build up a lifestyle that doesn't feel forced. It just feels like *you.* And that's the goal, right? To create a way of living that supports your health without constantly feeling like you're swimming upstream.

Staying motivated can be challenging, but finding joy in the journey makes all the difference. Celebrate your wins, no matter how small, and remember why you started. Each day is a new opportunity to grow, learn, and thrive.

By weaving the principles of The 100-50 Method into your daily life, you're not just building habits, you're creating a lifestyle that leads to lasting change.

Real Women, Real Wins

Here's Sandy's story. She is close to her goal and steadily still losing by building healthy habits with The 100-50 Method.

> "I love The 100-50 Method. Honestly, it's the only plan/diet/lifestyle change I've been able to stick with. It's realistic and will be easy for me to sustain. I'm grateful!

I just looked back through my calendar, and in the last nine weeks, I have lost two pounds each week. Just eighteen pounds to my goal! I don't think I could have gotten this far without all the information here! I love that I have protein and fats to count instead of calories. It has taught me how to eat in a way that is sustainable! I'm so grateful!

I love how Aimee & Erica have made this program so easy to understand! As a busy working mom of twin eleven-year-olds, I appreciate that this program is not complicated and is something I can easily incorporate into my life. I enjoy the Instagram reels explaining how this program works, sharing recipes, and giving reminders to get some squats or walks in. In addition to IG, I like the personal connection on The 100-50 Method Facebook group. It's a great space to read the program material, watch Aimee's IG videos, ask questions, celebrate one another's successes, and support/encourage one another.

The 100-50 program materials and information on IG and FB have helped me select excellent protein choices and great healthy fat options and add foods that help with satiety. One of the most important things Aimee shares is to do your food journaling the night before. When you are prepared, it's so

much easier to stay right on track. This reminder has stuck with me, and I usually prepare my whole day's food choices the night before. I'm feeling so positive about how this program has already impacted my life in such a positive way. Now, I am looking forward to a continued healthy lifestyle for many years to come!"
—Sandi P.

It's those small, daily habits that truly shape our journey—***tiny actions*** that snowball into incredible ***transformation***.

Your Forty Fix Era Is Here

You've made it to the end of this book, and we just want to take a moment to acknowledge how far you've come and celebrate the effort you've put in. This wasn't just about reading through nutrition tips or diving into hormone talk. It was about deciding that your health matters. **That YOU matter.** And that you're ready to make the changes you deserve.

When we first started this journey, we were tired. Tired of feeling like our bodies were broken. Tired of hearing, "That's just what happens in your forties." Tired of being told to "move more and eat less" when that just wasn't working. Tired of searching for answers that never came. But the truth is, our bodies weren't broken. They were just asking for support. They were begging us to tune in instead of tune out. To nourish instead of restrict. To fuel instead of deprive. And that shift? That's what became The 100-50 Method and ultimately *The Forty Fix*.

This isn't a plan you follow for thirty days and then drop like all the rest. **This is a method that becomes a mindset.** A new way of doing life, where energy, confidence, and clarity become your new normal. One where you stop spinning in cycles of restriction and start living in rhythms of nourishment. One where your habits support your health without stealing your joy.

Whether you're here to lose weight, balance hormones, improve energy, or simply feel like yourself again, this method meets you where you are. It flexes with your life, honors your real-world responsibilities, and reminds you that change doesn't have to feel like a full-time job. It can be simple. It can be doable. And it can feel really good.

You now understand the "why" behind everything: Why protein and healthy fats matter. Why blood sugar stability is the foundation for fat loss and hormone balance. Why three meals a day work better than endless grazing. Why GLP-1 plays a powerful role in hunger, metabolism, and weight loss. Why movement doesn't have to be extreme to be effective. Why habit stacking and food journaling change the game. This isn't just information; it's ***transformation*** **waiting to happen.**

Maybe right now, you're still figuring it out. Maybe you've had some great days and some messy ones. That's okay. We've been there too. Progress isn't linear, and perfection isn't the goal. The goal is to keep showing up. To keep choosing the next nourishing step, even when life is loud and complicated. To keep giving yourself grace on the hard days, and a high five on the days you feel unstoppable.

Our hope is that this book has shown you that taking care of yourself doesn't have to be hard. It doesn't have to be all-consuming. And it definitely doesn't have to be confusing. **The power is in the simplicity.** You're not counting calories, obsessing over macros, or starving your way to success. You're adding in. You're supporting your hormones. You're making decisions that align with the version of you that feels vibrant and alive.

And here's the best part: You're not doing this alone. There is an entire community of women walking this path with you. Women cheering you on, sharing their wins, posting their food journals, swapping recipes, and reminding you that, yes, it's absolutely possible to feel good again. If you haven't already, come find us. Come be part of something that's so much bigger than a "program." Because **this is a movement, and *we want you in it.***

We created The 100-50 Method because we wanted to feel good in our own skin again. What we didn't expect was how much better life gets when you do. How everything (from your sleep, to your confidence, to how you show up for your partner or your kids or your job) shifts. Because when women feel good, we show up fully. We lead. We create. We build meaningful lives. We change the world.

That is what *The Forty Fix* is all about: fixing it in your favor so you can live the life you have to the fullest.

So here's to your next chapter. The one where you're not held back by fatigue, cravings, or stubborn weight. The one where you wake up with energy, eat with purpose, move with intention, and live in a body that feels like home again. You've got the tools, the knowledge, and, most importantly, the M.E.T.H.O.D.

Now go live it. And keep fixing it in your favor every single day.

We're rooting for you every step of the way.

With so much love,
Aimee & Erica

The

End

Appendix

Aimee: 7-Day Food Journal

Here's my food journal from this past week (where P stands for protein and HF for healthy fat). It was a full, non-stop week—lots of kid activities, all five heading in different directions, and plenty of time spent in the car.

You'll notice a few days where dinner happened on the go, between pick-ups and drop-offs, and I opted for a protein smoothie. If I'm home for lunch or dinner, I often have a few bites of sauerkraut or some pickles while I'm prepping my food to get my GLP-1 secretion going. This is usually when I have ACV as well. I also have a liquid collagen I drink at the end of my lunch, which adds another 5 grams of protein to my daily total (but I leave it out of my food journal so I get to 100g or more without it).

Day 1

Breakfast – Protein Smoothie

Protein powder – 24g P & 6g HF

2 tbsp chia seeds – 4g P & 8g HF

2 tbsp ground flaxseeds – 3g P & 5g HF

Total – 31g P & 19g HF

Lunch – Chicken Salad Boats

Lettuce boats with chicken, shredded carrots, and cottage cheese (& homemade mustard/lemon juice dressing)

Chicken – 39g P & 22g HF

1/2 cup cottage cheese – 12g P & 3g HF

Total – 52g P & 25g HF

Dinner – Shrimp Sheet Pan

Tomatoes, asparagus, garlic, and spices

Shrimp – 39g P & 3g HF

Olive oil – 14g HF

Total – 39g P & 17g HF

Daily total – 122g P & 61g HF

Day 2

Breakfast – Protein Smoothie

Protein powder – 24g P & 6g HF

2 tbsp chia seeds – 4g P & 8g HF

2 tbsp ground flaxseeds – 3g P & 5g HF

Total – 31g P & 19g HF

Lunch – Green + Grains Bowl from Cava

With falafel + extra protein grilled chicken (lentils for my grain)

SuperGreens, black lentils, red pepper hummus, tzatziki, crazy feta, grilled chicken, falafel, pickled onions, tomato + onion, salt-brined pickles, Persian cucumber, crumbled feta

Total – 40g P & 30g HF

Dinner – Taco Bowl

Ground beef with tomatoes & veggies & cheese

Total – 34g P & 9g HF

Daily total – 105g P & 58g HF

Day 3

Breakfast – Protein Smoothie

Protein powder – 24g P & 6g HF

2 tbsp chia seeds – 4g P & 8g HF

2 tbsp ground flaxseeds – 3g P & 5g HF

Total – 31g P & 19g HF

Lunch – Egg Scramble & Broccoli

1/4 cup cottage cheese – 6g P & 3g HF

4 eggs – 24g P & 20g HF

Total – 30g P & 23g HF

Dinner – Salmon & Asparagus

Salmon – 44g P & 15g HF

Daily total – 105g P & 57g HF

Day 4

Breakfast – Protein Smoothie

Protein powder – 24g P & 6g HF

2 tbsp chia seeds – 4g P & 8g HF

2 tbsp ground flaxseeds – 3g P & 5g HF

Total – 31g P & 19g HF

Lunch – Veggie & Black Bean Salad

Spinach, arugula, carrots, bell peppers, sauerkraut

1/2 cup black beans – 8g P

3 hard-boiled eggs – 18g P & 15g HF

1/2 cup cottage cheese – 12g P & 3g HF

1/2 avocado – 2g P & 14g HF

Total – 40g P & 32g HF

Dinner – Protein Smoothie & Greek Yogurt Parfait (on the run)

Protein powder – 24g & 6g HF

Greek yogurt 3/4 cup – 16g P

2 tbsp chia seeds – 4g P & 8g HF

Blueberries & raspberries

Total – 44g P & 14g HF

Daily total – 115g P & 65g HF

Day 5

Breakfast – Protein Smoothie

Protein powder – 24g P & 6g HF

2 tbsp chia seeds – 4g P & 8g HF

2 tbsp ground flaxseeds – 3g P & 5g HF

Total – 31g P & 19g HF

Lunch – Egg Scramble & Broccoli

¼ cup cottage cheese – 6g P & 3g HF

4 eggs – 24g P & 20g HF

Total – 30g P & 23g HF

Dinner – Chicken Sheet Pan

Carrots, broccoli, bell peppers, onions, garlic

Olive oil – 14g HF

Chicken – 39g P

Total – 39g P & 14g HF

Daily total – 100g P & 56g HF

Day 6

Breakfast – Eggs & Yogurt Parfait

1/4 cup cottage cheese – 6g P & 3g HF

4 eggs – 24g P & 20g HF

&

Greek yogurt 3/4 cup – 16g p

2 tbsp chia seeds – 4g P & 8g HF

Blueberries & raspberries

Total – 50g P & 31g HF

Lunch – Veggie & Black Bean Salad

Spinach, arugula, carrots, bell peppers, sauerkraut

1/2 cup black beans – 8g P

1/2 cup cottage cheese – 12g P & 3g HF

2 hard-boiled eggs – 12g P & 10g HF

Total – 32g P & 13g HF

Dinner – Salmon & Asparagus

Salmon – 44g P & 15g HF

Daily total – 126g P & 59g HF

Day 7

Breakfast – Protein Smoothie

Protein powder – 24g P & 6g HF

2 tbsp chia seeds – 4g P & 8g HF

2 tbsp ground flaxseeds – 3g P & 5g HF

Total – 31g P & 19g HF

Lunch – Salade Niçoise

Lettuce, tomatoes, carrots with:

3 hard-boiled eggs – 18g P & 15g HF

1 packet of tuna (mixed with Dijon mustard) – 17g p

1/2 avocado – 2g P & 14g HF

Total – 37g P & 29g HF

Dinner – Protein Smoothie & Greek Yogurt Parfait (on the run)

Protein powder – 24g & 6g HF

Greek yogurt 3/4 cup – 16g p

2 tbsp chia seeds – 4g P & 8g HF

Blueberries & raspberries

Total – 44g P & 14g HF

Daily total – 112g P & 62g HF

Erica: 7-Day Food Journal

Around my house, meals are simple and doable. Nothing fancy, just real food that fuels us and fits into the rhythm of everyday life. I'm not trying to reinvent the wheel or make separate meals for everyone at the table.

We eat together as a family whenever we can, and I've found little ways to adjust my plate without complicating dinner for everyone else. While I might tweak my portion or skip the bun, my plate still looks a whole lot like everyone else's.

Day 1

Breakfast – Scrambled Eggs Plate

3 scrambled eggs

Turkey sausage (3 links)

Sautéed spinach in olive oil

Total – 32g P & 22g HF

Lunch – Chicken Bowl

Grilled chicken breast (6 oz)

Quinoa

Mixed greens

Olive oil vinaigrette

Total – 34g P & 14g HF

Dinner – Sheet Pan Chicken & Veggies

Chicken thighs

Bell peppers

Carrots

Onions

Olive oil

Roasted sweet potato

Total – 35g P & 14g HF

Daily Total – 101g P & 50g HF

Day 2

Breakfast – Yogurt Bowl

Greek yogurt (1.5 cups)

Chia seeds

Almonds

Blueberries

Total – 32g P & 18g HF

Lunch – Tuna Salad

Tuna (2 cans)

Olive oil mayo

Celery

Pickles

Ezekiel toast

Total – 38g P & 20g HF

Dinner – Burger Night

6 oz lean ground beef patty

Lettuce wrap (no bun)

Tomato

Avocado

Baked sweet potato fries

Total – 30g P & F 13g HF

Daily Total – 100g P & 51g HF

Day 3

Breakfast – Protein Smoothie

Protein powder

1 tbsp peanut butter

Almond milk

Banana

Flaxseed

Total – 35g P & 15g HF

Lunch – Turkey and Hummus Wrap

Whole grain wrap

6 oz turkey breast

2 tbsp hummus

Spinach

Total – 35g P & 12g HF

Dinner – Chicken Stir Fry

Chicken breast

Broccoli

Bell peppers

Snap peas

Sesame oil

Brown rice

Total – 32g P & 23g HF

Daily Total – 102g P & 50g HF

Day 4

Breakfast – Veggie Omelet

3 eggs

Mushrooms

Spinach

Feta

1/2 avocado

Total – 28g P & 22g HF

Lunch – Leftover Stir Fry

Leftover chicken stir fry (from day 3 Dinner)

Extra chicken

Total – 36g P & 14g HF

Dinner – Sheet Pan Salmon & Veggies

Salmon fillet

Asparagus

Olive oil

Quinoa

Total – 36g P & 14g HF

Daily Total – 100g P & 50g HF

Day 5

Breakfast – Yogurt Bowl

Skyr Greek yogurt (plain, 1.5 cups)

Walnuts (1 tbsp)

Strawberries

Total – 30g P & 15g HF

Lunch – Chicken Caesar Salad

6 oz grilled chicken

Romaine

Parmesan

Primal Kitchen Caesar dressing

Total – 35g P & 20g HF

Dinner – Meatballs & Zoodles

Turkey Meatballs (about 6 medium meatballs)

Zucchini noodles

Marinara

Olive oil drizzle

Total – 35g P & 15g HF

Daily Total – 100g P & 50g HF

Day 6

Breakfast – Protein Smoothie

Protein powder

Chia seeds

Almond butter

Almond milk

Frozen berries

Total – 34g P & 15g HF

Lunch – Egg Salad

3 eggs

Avocado mayo

Grilled chicken breast (4 oz)

Mixed greens

Total – 35g P & 20g HF

Dinner – Steak Fajita Sheet Pan

Steak

Bell peppers

Onions

Olive oil

Taco seasoning

Black beans

Total – 34g P & 15g HF

Daily Total – 103g P & 50g HF

Day 7

Breakfast – Protein Chia Pudding

Protein powder

Chia seeds

Pumpkin seeds

Total – 30g P & 20g HF

Lunch – Grilled chicken wrap

6 oz chicken

Whole wheat wrap

Greek yogurt ranch

Lettuce

Total – 34g P & 15g HF

Dinner – Baked Chicken Parmesan

Chicken breast

Marinara

Mozzarella

Roasted broccoli & cauliflower

Olive oil drizzle

Total – 36g P & 15g HF

Daily Total – 100g P & 50g HF

Blank 7-Day Food Journal

Here's a Blank 7-Day Food Journal so that you can track your protein and healthy fats throughout the day.

Think of these pages as a mirror for your journey. The more consistent you are in writing things down, the more clarity you'll gain about what's working for your body. Some days will feel effortless, and other days may feel messy . . . but every day you show up here, you're proving to yourself that your health and energy matter.

Use this journal as often as you can, not to chase perfection, but to create awareness. Awareness turns into habits, habits turn into results, and results turn into the confident, energized version of you that you've been craving. This is your daily invitation to keep fixing it in your favor.

Day 1

Breakfast –

Total –

Lunch –

Total –

Dinner –

Total –

Daily total –

Day 2

Breakfast –

Total –

Lunch –

Total –

Dinner –

Total –

Daily total –

Day 3

Breakfast –

Total –

Lunch –

Total –

Dinner –

Total –

Daily total –

Day 4

Breakfast –

Total –

Lunch –

Total –

Dinner –

Total –

Daily total –

Day 5

Breakfast –

Total –

Lunch –

Total –

Dinner –

Total –

Daily total –

Day 6

Breakfast –

Total –

Lunch –

Total –

Dinner –

Total –

Daily total –

Day 7

Breakfast –

Total –

Lunch –

Total –

Dinner –

Total –

Daily total –

Printed in Dunstable, United Kingdom

68847235R00089